Journeys
with the
Cancer
Conqueror

Journeys

with the

Cancer Conqueror

Mobilizing Mind and Spirit

✦

Greg Anderson

Foreword by Abigail Van Buren

Andrews McMeel Publishing

Kansas City

99 00 01 02 03 RDH 10 9 8 7 6 5 4 3 2 1

www.andrewsmcmeel.com

Library of Congress Cataloging-in-Publication Data

Anderson, Greg, 1947–
    Journeys with cancer conqueror : mobilizing mind and spirit / Greg Anderson. —Rev. ed.
        p. cm.
    Previously published under the title: The cancer conqueror.
    ISBN 0-7407-0020-0
    1. Cancer—Psychosomatic aspects. 2. Cancer—Psychological aspects. I. Anderson, Greg, 1947– Cancer conqueror. II. Title.
RC262.A66 1999
616.99'4'0019—dc21   99-22165
                                                   CIP

ATTENTION: SCHOOLS AND BUSINESSES

Andrews McMeel books are available at quantity discounts with bulk purchase for educational, business, or sales promotional use. For information, please write to: Special Sales Department, Andrews McMeel Publishing, 4520 Main Street, Kansas City, Missouri 64111.

With gratitude to my wife, Linda,
and our daughter, Erica.
Thank you for your constant love and support.
You, too, are Cancer Conquerors.

❧ *Contents* ❧

❧ *Foreword* ❧

Every day I receive heartbreaking letters from people who have lost all hope because they have just been diagnosed with cancer. They feel powerless, frightened, and without direction. Some of them resign themselves to the inevitable—but they shouldn't. People *can* conquer cancer—they *can* recover.

When Greg Anderson wrote *The Cancer Conqueror* he shared his own successful mental "battle plan" with which he fought metastasized lung cancer after being given only thirty days to live. I was gratified to play a part in bringing its timeless and inspiring message to the attention of my readers, because it was the first time I had seen a book that gave people who suffer from cancer—and those who love them—a message of real hope. Since then, it has helped hundreds of thousands of cancer patients.

Now, from the same author, comes an even more powerful tool for helping cancer patients establish an active role in their recovery. Many writers feel compelled to tell others what to think and do. With this book, *Journeys with the Cancer Conqueror: Mobilizing Mind and Spirit*, Greg Anderson allows us to see for *ourselves* what we are thinking. This helps cancer patients to tap deeply into their spirits and uncover the incredible healing power of hope by realizing, "I am stronger and possess more resources than I thought!" This helps the patient to evolve from barely surviving to living in a state of grace, able to celebrate each sacred moment. This is truly a powerful message in a most remarkable book.

This much I know to be true: Reading books can change lives. And this book will change yours, by revealing a secret: When you discover you have cancer, you *do* have a choice—you can prepare to die or you can prepare to live. It is exactly when you make choices about your life and your treatment that your cancer no longer controls you.

If you or someone you love is facing the crisis of cancer, *Journeys with the Cancer Conqueror* is a must-read. Pick it up and begin living its message today.

Abigail Van Buren
"Dear Abby"

❧ *Preface* ❧

Believe it. It is possible to survive, even thrive, following a cancer diagnosis.

I lovingly write this book from the cancer patient's perspective. I am a survivor of metastatic lung cancer. In 1984, a surgeon told me, "Greg, the tiger is out of the cage. Your cancer has come roaring back. I would give you about thirty days to live."

Since that time, I have worked directly with more than 15,000 cancer survivors. This much has become increasingly and abundantly clear to me: The body's healing capacity is directly linked to one's mental and spiritual well-being. Embracing healthy beliefs and attitudes, learning to effectively resolve emotional distress, and moving in the direction of greater joy and gratitude all have a direct impact on our physical health.

Cancer is a message to change. And those changes are desirable. Read this book. Make the changes. Live this message. You, too, will become a cancer conqueror.

Greg Anderson
Hershey, Pennsylvania, U.S.A.
August 1999

Journeys
with the
Cancer
Conqueror

❧ 1 ❧

Cancer Conquerors Search

Once there was a man who received a diagnosis of cancer.

The man did not want cancer. He wanted to be well, to be disease-free. He wanted to live a full and happy life.

To him cancer was a frightening enemy. And the fear it brought was a sinking feeling in his stomach that death was just about to overtake him. *Was this all there was to life?* There was so much left undone, so much that might have been. Maybe that was the worst part of all.

Why me? He took care of himself throughout his fifty-plus years. Oh, he didn't always eat exactly the right foods and sometimes didn't get enough sleep. But certainly he never abused his body. Several of his friends were much worse by comparison.

And what did all this mean medically? It was bad

enough to think that there might be only a short life span ahead. But maybe even worse, a long life of incapacitation. That would be unthinkable.

His mind raced. *How could this happen to me? I'm losing control.* It all seemed so frightening, so futile.

In the meantime, the man looked for someone who had already walked the same path, someone who had found the answer and who might be willing to share his or her experience.

First the man began asking the medical team. His family doctor referred him to a number of medical specialists, but the person the man trusted the most was his oncologist. This doctor was highly respected. He was directing the man's treatment—a plan that included a surgeon and other professionals.

The man inquired about his chances for successful recovery.

"I rate your chances good," replied the oncologist. "We have every reason to believe that surgery removed the entire tumor and that radiation will act as a double check."

This was all reassuring. But the man was still consumed by a gnawing sense of fear. So many more questions remained unanswered.

He wished he could talk to someone who had been through a similar experience.

Once he found a long-term survivor, but she looked as if she might die any minute. Even though she had survived for five years—the standard "you are cured" time frame— her quality of life was less than desirable. He wasn't looking for poor life quality.

The man knew that for his sake, as well as for the people around him, he had to find his answers soon.

Then he remembered a co-worker who, several years ago, had lived through cancer. And the interesting thing about his friend's experience was that the cancer journey seemed to have changed her much for the better. Not only was this woman's cancer under control but she seemed to be leading a new life, a better life than ever before.

Maybe I should talk to her right away, thought the man. When he called his friend's home, one of the children said her parents were on a trip and wouldn't return for another week. Then she certainly must be doing well, decided the man.

He asked the friend's daughter, "Do you know what doctor your mother saw?"

"No," she replied, "I don't know the doctor. But I do know that she spent the most time with the Cancer Conqueror."

"The Cancer Conqueror?" asked the man.

"Yes," answered the daughter. "That's the affectionate name we gave to a woman and a group of her friends who taught my mother and our family about cancer. We learned that people can conquer cancer and, in doing so, may even cure it."

The man felt a positive, supportive attitude from the girl when she asked, "Do you have cancer?"

"Yes," said the man. "How can I get in touch with the Cancer Conqueror?"

He took down a telephone number, thanked the daughter, and smiled. "How is your mother now?" he asked.

"Never been better," said the daughter. "Cancer has changed our whole family's life, all for the better."

"Thank you," said the man as he hung up.

This was more than a little strange. Cancer making changes for the better in the life of an entire family? That was a little difficult to believe. Yet the daughter sounded so sure. Maybe there was something to be learned from this terrible thing called cancer after all.

The man called the Cancer Conqueror that same morning, and they made an appointment for the following afternoon. He couldn't wait to meet the Cancer Conqueror.

2

Cancer Conquerors Take Responsibility

From the moment the man arrived at the home of the Cancer Conqueror, he felt an excitement and warmth that he could not explain. And the feeling was reinforced when the Cancer Conqueror answered the door with a warm greeting and an easy smile.

So this was the Cancer Conqueror! She had such an approachable manner about her. And her smile—it seemed to come as much from her eyes as from her mouth.

They made their way to a large patio overlooking a beautifully landscaped backyard garden. Chilled juice had been prepared and was awaiting them at the table. They pulled up comfortable chairs, and the Cancer Conqueror asked the man to describe briefly his disease and the prognosis.

Then the Cancer Conqueror asked, "Do you have a high level of confidence in your medical team?"

"Yes," said the man, "I believe they are very knowledgeable and that they have the latest in available technology."

"Excellent. The basis for my recovery also started with a fine medical team. I had a great deal of confidence in their abilities and in them as individuals also. But I insisted that they share all information with me in terms I could understand. And I wanted explanations for each and every test. I had to be part of every treatment decision. What I was really doing was taking personal responsibility for my health—personal responsibility for getting well."

"I'm not sure what you mean," said the man. "What is personal responsibility for getting well?"

The Cancer Conqueror leaned forward and looked directly and emphatically into the man's eyes.

"Personal responsibility for getting well, for conquering cancer, is one of the most important principles of the entire cancer journey. If you choose this path—the cancer conqueror path—personal responsibility will come up again and again. It is one of those cornerstone principles that supports everything else.

"Personal responsibility for health means refusing to be a victim. It means participating in recovery by recognizing and changing self-destructive beliefs and behavior. Personal responsibility for health means believing 'I am in charge of my cancer. My cancer is not in charge of me.'

"And personal responsibility has simple logic to it. The medical team, no matter how esteemed, functions largely in the role of mechanics. They are trained in cell biology. They can operate and prescribe treatments, but they are not

❧❧

I am in charge of my cancer.
My cancer is not
in charge of me.

❧❧

responsible for our life or ultimately our health. We are! Nobody can get well for us. We have to do it for ourselves.

"Selecting a medical team in which we have a high level of confidence is our first responsibility after diagnosis. But once they are in place, our attention must also focus on the role of mind and spirit in this journey."

"Mind and spirit?" asked the man. "I have a physical problem, not an emotional one."

The Cancer Conqueror nodded. Her smile said she understood.

"When I encountered cancer, I instinctively knew that this was not just an experience on a physical level. I knew that my mind and spirit had a central role to play. Personal responsibility meant that if I was to live a full and healthy life, whatever the length, that decision rested not with my doctors but with me. I also realized that once my medical team made its contribution, it was my job to discover and use all my healing potential. This perspective leads beyond the body to the mind and the spirit."

"Are you saying that cancer is more than just a physical disease?"

❧❧

Cancer is more than
just a physical disease.

❧❧

"Yes! That's exactly what I'm saying. You certainly have a physical problem. It is an abnormality with your cells. But that's just one facet, one level of the problem. As a living human being, you are much more than your body. You are also your mind and your spirit. That means you can bring these resources, as well as the biological, to the solution. The members of the medical team will do all they can to help the body. If you will support them with good nutrition, exercise, and rest, the physical portion of the journey will be in place."

"Okay," said the man. "I'll do those things. But I'm not sure about the mind and the spirit. Can I learn?"

The Cancer Conqueror stopped and smiled. If this person really meant that question, there was hope. With an attitude of open curiosity about the mind and spirit, much could happen. The man stood an excellent chance of being a Cancer Conqueror.

"Come, let's walk," said the Cancer Conqueror. "Let me share some of my personal story."

As they walked to the gate, the man sensed that he was about to hear something special. He was ready to listen and learn.

"It was breast cancer," said the Cancer Conqueror. "The

doctor put his hand on my shoulder and said that surgery was the only answer. The breast would have to be removed.

"They performed surgery, but six months later a growth started protruding from my neck. Again, surgery. It was malignant. The cancer had now spread, and they could not operate. The surgeon closed the incision, ordered radiation therapy, and told me to get my affairs in order. According to statistics, I had a year, maybe a little more, to live."

The man was astonished. "My chances are much better than that. How did you do it?"

The Cancer Conqueror stopped and leaned against the fence.

"After my second surgery, I was frightened and had virtually lost all hope. I believed the doctors' prognosis. The fear of my life coming to a sudden end paralyzed me.

"I was sitting on the couch looking at my daughter playing with a doll. I suddenly thought, I will not live to see her grow up. It was the lowest point. I don't know of any point of deeper despair. Tears filled my eyes. It was over. The next words that came out were full of rage and anger and fear. 'Oh God, what can I do?'

"But somehow through the tears, a different thought came. It was as if someone was saying, 'You may not be given long to live, but live as long as you are given.'

❧❧

You may not be given long to live,

but live as long as you are given.

❧❧

"I discovered a seed of hope in that thought, a seed I knew needed special care and attention. 'Live as long as you are given.' It was a seed that provided sustenance for me during the countless down times. I knew that every day I had to rededicate myself to living that one day for all it was worth. Looking over at my daughter, I thought, I may not be here to love her tomorrow. But I am here today. How can I show her my love now?

"Love now. This is the core of conquering cancer."

"It sounds so simplistic," said the man. "Isn't there more?"

"Much more," agreed the Cancer Conqueror. "This is merely the tip of a powerful transformational discovery. But living today, doing the best I could to make love my aim, here and now, held a tremendous message of hope and healing for me. It changed not only my health but my entire life. That same message has embodied healing for thousands of others. And I believe it can do the same for you.

"If you want to take this journey, your first assignment will be to visit three different people over the next three weeks. You will learn about three Cancer Conqueror principles:

❧ Believe

❧ Resolve

❧ Live

"If you complete the assignment, come back and we will talk about why this works and look at the real benefits of conquering cancer. Is this something you would like to do?"

It all seemed too simple, as if there were some sort of formula to use and then everything would be okay. The man wasn't sure he understood all the Cancer Conqueror had said, but he heard himself saying, "Okay, what do I have to lose?"

The Cancer Conqueror stopped and looked at the man with that now-familiar smile that came from her eyes. "All you have to lose," she said, "is your fear, anger, and guilt. I'll set up the first appointment for you. Over the weekend, give thought to your personal responsibility for getting well. Remember: You are in charge of your response to cancer!"

❈ Readers' Choice ❈

Our story continues on page 31. Before you go on, you may want to complete the following exercises. They are designed to heighten your sense of personal control, a critical ingredient in your journey to wellness.

❧ PERSONAL RESPONSIBILITY: ❧ GAINING A SENSE OF CONTROL

The degree to which a patient takes personal responsibility for his or her own actions and feelings in response to a cancer diagnosis is a crucially important determinant of the course of an illness. I urge you to take responsibility for your proactive response, beginning immediately.

Awareness and choice are the twin pillars that support personal responsibility. We increase awareness through our personal research and education, becoming eager students, ready to learn everything we can about our diagnosis and range of treatment options. From this knowledge base, we exercise fully informed consent to treatments and make intentional choices in our physical, emotional, and spiritual lifestyles.

In your cancer journey, the power of personal responsibility is stupendous; its implications are massive.

Recognize first the potential negative consequences; if we don't give mindful attention to our diagnosis, treatment, diet, exercise, emotional outlook, and spiritual choices, we will surely not respond to cancer with optimum capacity. Ignore our personal responsibility and we fail to implement a comprehensive recovery program.

The good news is that the personal responsibility coin has two sides. Just as less-than-mindful attention will contribute to a less-than-optimal response, a fully mindful response holds the promise of direct health benefits. We have the power to become aware of and make changes in our beliefs and behavior. It is as simple, and as complex, as changing our thinking.

When we assume personal responsibility for our choices, we have the ability to change our every experience of cancer.

Having experienced both sides of this coin, I have no doubt of personal responsibility's significant power. After my cancerous left lung was removed, I quickly reverted to my previous behaviors. My diet consisted of too much high-fat fast food. My exercise program was sporadic at best. I lived an adrenaline-charged, workaholic life. I demonstrated an overly critical and disagreeable spirit.

I believe those personal choices greatly contributed to my return to the hospital a short four months later. It was then discovered that the cancer was throughout my lymph system. The surgeon said, "Greg, the tiger is out of the cage. Your cancer has come roaring back. I would give you about thirty days to live."

There's nothing like bad news to either paralyze or energize. The thirty-day prognosis focused my attention and energy. I felt I had two ways to turn. One was to give in to the despair and prepare to die. The other, even though it held no promise of success, was to participate fully in an effort to get well again. I chose the latter.

Today, I have come to realize the vitally important role each patient plays in his or her recovery. Central to success is assuming personal responsibility for proper diet and appropriate exercise. Stress management has a key supportive role and deserves to be understood and implemented by the serious wellness student. So do beliefs and attitudes, resolution of emotional conflict and hostility, plus capturing a sense of joy. And adopting a more spiritual focus on life may be the most important recovery tool of all.

Nobody can accomplish these tasks for us. Nobody can get well for us. Others can help, of course. But in the final analysis, we must walk the wellness path for ourselves. We stand personally accountable for this journey.

Where do you rate yourself on personal responsibility? I invite you to conduct an important self-test. Gauge your level of personal responsibility by taking a searching personal inventory based on the following queries.

Examine Your Level of Personal Responsibility

Consider each statement. Indicate your level of agreement by circling the relative value from 10 to 1, 10 indicating that you strongly agree, 1 that you strongly disagree.

❧ I am in charge of my experience of cancer.

Strongly agree		Somewhat agree		Not certain either way		Somewhat disagree		Strongly disagree	
10	9	8	7	6	5	4	3	2	1

Thought Starters: What does "being in charge" actually mean to me? What is within my sphere of influence? Is "control" really possible, or even preferable, for me?

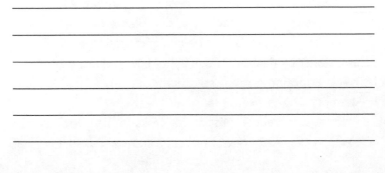

_____

_____

_____

_____

_____

_____

_____

_____

❧ **Getting well again is not just a matter of genetics and medical treatment.**

Strongly agree		Somewhat agree		Not certain either way		Somewhat disagree		Strongly disagree	
10	9	8	7	6	5	4	3	2	1

Thought Starter: What must I personally contribute to the process beyond selecting a treatment program?

_____

_____

_____

_____

_____

_____

_____

❧ **My personal efforts do make a difference in my recovery.**

Strongly agree		Somewhat agree		Not certain either way		Somewhat disagree		Strongly disagree
10	9	8	7	6	5	4	3	2	1

Thought Starter: When I think of myself as making a difference, what do I picture myself doing?

_____

_____

_____

✖ **I have the ability to discriminate between what is controllable and what is uncontrollable in the cancer journey.**

Strongly agree		Somewhat agree		Not certain either way		Somewhat disagree		Strongly disagree
10	9	8	7	6	5	4	3	2	1

Thought Starters: How can I most effectively control my fears? How can I create a calm and quiet healing environment?

_____

_____

_____

_____

_____

_____

_____

_____

_____

_____

_____

_____

_____

_____

❧ My mind and spirit have a central role in my recovery.

Strongly agree		Somewhat agree		Not certain either way		Somewhat disagree		Strongly disagree	
10	9	8	7	6	5	4	3	2	1

Thought Starters: Is my state of mind and spirit most often positive or negative? What can I do to nurture a more positive mental and spiritual outlook?

_____

_____

_____

_____

_____

_____

_____

_____

_____

_____

_____

❧ Registering my emotions using "I feel . . ." instead of "You make me feel . . ." brings me empowerment.

Strongly agree		Somewhat agree		Not certain either way		Somewhat disagree		Strongly disagree	
10	9	8	7	6	5	4	3	2	1

Thought Starters: Do I fully understand the statement "Cancer doesn't make me fearful (angry/guilty), I make me fearful (angry/guilty)"? How do I make myself fearful (angry/guilty)? Can I truly master my fear (anger/guilt)?

❧ **When I have moments of feeling helpless, victimized, and depressed, I have ready resources that empower me.**

Strongly agree		Somewhat agree		Not certain either way		Somewhat disagree		Strongly disagree	
10	9	8	7	6	5	4	3	2	1

Thought Starter: List the people, places, and things you can turn to to lift your mind and spirit—without fail.

_____

_____

_____

_____

_____

_____

_____

_____

_____

_____

_____

_____

_____

_____

_____

_____

❧ I possess considerable power to create the life and well-being I desire.

Strongly agree		Somewhat agree		Not certain either way		Somewhat disagree		Strongly disagree	
10	9	8	7	6	5	4	3	2	1

Thought Starter: When I think of myself as well, what is the image I carry in my mind?

_____

_____

_____

_____

_____

_____

_____

_____

_____

_____

_____

_____

_____

_____

_____

_____

_____

Reflect on your answers and the level of intensity surrounding each belief.

For the Advanced Wellness Student

When people disown personal responsibility, it can often be seen in their language. A person who says, "That doctor makes me so mad," is throwing responsibility for his anger onto his doctor. A breast cancer patient who says, "I prefer to have my surgery during the second half of my menstrual cycle," is taking responsibility for her own needs in a more direct way.*

Accusatory "you" statements can be signs that patients and family members are blaming others rather than setting out to solve their own problems or to make their feelings and needs known. Many times this happens because the person does not take responsibility, or feel permitted, to say, "I don't like what is happening in my life at this time." Instead, the words come out as "You (or the doctor, or the nurse, or the receptionist) are making me upset."

Examine your own behavior. "You" statements indicate that the speaker holds someone else responsible for his happiness and well-being. The speaker thus gives up considerable personal control. He depends on other people to be aware of his needs and fulfill them. Someone else is given the duty of making his personal choices. If things don't work out satisfactorily, someone else gets the blame.

*There is mounting evidence that premenopausal women have fewer recurrences when breast cancer surgery is performed in the luteal phase, days 14–30, of the menstrual cycle. Ask your physician.

Cancer patients who choose the journey to wellness tend to make "I" statements that express their own needs, feelings, likes, and dislikes. This does not mean the patients are without support or "go it alone." Instead, there is a clear understanding among the patient, the health care team, and the primary support team that each individual is responsible for determining how he or she will respond to cancer in his or her own life.

Become aware of your own level of personal responsibility. Analyze your responses to the following queries. Are they true or false? How or why might you be reacting that way? List several ways you might change.

❧ Cancer doesn't make me fearful, I make me fearful.

_____

_____

_____

_____

_____

_____

_____

_____

_____

_____

_____

_____

_____

_____

_____

_____

❧ **The doctor doesn't make me angry, I make me angry.**

_____

_____

_____

_____

_____

_____

_____

_____

_____

_____

_____

_____

_____

_____

_____

_____

_____

❧ **My husband (wife/partner/child/friend) doesn't make me feel guilty, I make me feel guilty.**

_____

_____

_____

_____

_____

_____

_____

_____

_____

_____

_____

_____

❧ **What kinds of feelings about personal responsibility do these queries evoke? Does this task of personal responsibility seem to be too much for you? In what ways and areas?**

_____

_____

_____

Blame is one of the surest ways to stay mired in a problem. When we blame another person, we give away our power. The moment we become aware of and begin to understand this dynamic, we rise above the issue and take control of our responses.

Don't blame the past; it cannot be changed. Don't blame the fear of an unknown future; we shape our future by our current state of mind and spirit. Don't blame doctors or hospitals or health care insurers or parents or spouses. Whenever we blame someone or something else, we are not taking personal responsibility for ourselves.

Most important, don't blame or demand perfection from yourself. If you do, you will be miserable every waking moment. Don't blame. Instead, channel that energy into creating a place in your mind and spirit where you are well. Then live from that place.

❧ **Describe a state of mind in which you are physically, emotionally, and spiritually well. Dwell on that image and create it vividly in your mind. How can you make that mental place a reality?**

_____

_____

_____

_____

_____

_____

_____

_____

_____

_____

_____

_____

_____

_____

_____

_____

_____

_____

❧ Be Gentle ❧

Nurture yourself. After you complete these exercises, I suggest you take a break from your wellness work. Contemplate the important issues raised. Listen carefully to your inner wisdom; healing knocks softly. Return to the story after you have rested.

❧ 3 ❧

Cancer Conquerors Believe

The following Monday, the man found himself at a home just a few blocks from his own. He'd walked by here several times and remembered chuckling at the sign over the doorbell—LOVE SPOKEN HERE.

Now here he was, at this same house seeking answers to which he wasn't even sure he knew the questions. It seemed more than a little ironic.

An attractive woman opened the door. Her voice was pleasant. "Welcome, I'm Mary. I've looked forward to talking with you ever since the Cancer Conqueror called last week. She's quite a person, isn't she?" As she talked Mary led the man to a table where she had hot water and herb teas waiting for them.

"Yes, she is," said the man as he sat down. "Do you mind if I take notes?" he asked.

"That's great," said Mary. "When the Cancer Conqueror called, she said we should cover the area of beliefs. So let's get started. Our point of departure is to ask you a question. What do you think cancer means?"

"I'm not sure," said the man. "I know it is a serious illness that will probably end my life pretty quickly unless I do something about it. And the Cancer Conqueror said it was more than physical. To me cancer is the worst nightmare I've ever had to deal with."

Mary smiled. "Those are pretty common beliefs about cancer. Society has conditioned us to think negatively and fearfully about this disease. And while some of that conditioning can be good, it has resulted in harmful untruths like these:

- 🌿 Cancer means death.
- 🌿 Treatment options are limited and ineffective and have horrible side effects.
- 🌿 Once you contract cancer, there is nothing you can do to help yourself.

"The truth is that

- 🌿 Cancer may or may not mean death.
- 🌿 Treatment options are many and are becoming more effective, and side effects are less severe every day.
- 🌿 Once you contract cancer, there are many things you can do—physically, emotionally, and spiritually—to help yourself.

"The untruths lead to beliefs that result in despair. With despair there is no power. But the truths lead to hope. With hope there is significant power.

"What you choose to believe about cancer is crucial to your journey. Note how the truths match three belief areas—the disease itself, the treatment, and your role. Your beliefs about the disease, the treatment, and your role have incredible power over the outcome, and you can choose these beliefs."

The man could see why the Cancer Conqueror wanted him to meet Mary. She was forceful as she talked about beliefs. He actually held most of the negative beliefs Mary had mentioned.

"I want to believe the hopeful thoughts," admitted the man, "but I don't know if I can believe them immediately."

"Sometimes," said Mary, "beliefs don't change easily. Let's look at each one more closely. First, the disease itself. It is a fact; cancer is not synonymous with death. When I was diagnosed with breast cancer seven years ago, I thought I was going to die. Then I learned more about the disease. Cancer is actually cured in about half the cases. And now over 90 percent of the patients who have the type of cancer I had survive for five years. The fact is, cancer does not mean death. The truth is, it may or may not mean death."

The man was writing notes. Okay, that was certainly true. His cancer was not an automatic death sentence. That would be a positive belief he could keep. Just because he had cancer did not mean he was going to die. It was affirming to hear Mary say so.

Mary paused only long enough for him to have a sip of tea. "The treatments are next. What do you believe about treatments?" she asked.

The man paused. "I guess I feel they are probably not very effective. And when it comes to side effects, I'm afraid of all the horrible possibilities."

Mary had had a similar experience with her cancer journey. "I felt the same way when I started. My treatment was surgery followed by chemotherapy. I, too, heard only bad things about mastectomies. And chemotherapy—I believed it was a last-hope drug. But then the doctor gave me assurances. The surgery was highly effective. And the chemotherapy gave me a small statistical advantage, which I chose. The truth was that the treatment plan was very hopeful."

"And the side effects?" asked the man.

"I was fortunate," said Mary. "Just as I was beginning the chemotherapy sessions, I read about the psychological component of side effects. A research study tracked a group of people who were given sterile water injections instead of chemotherapy, and a third of them lost their hair anyway."

"I don't understand," said the man.

"The only explanation the researchers could give for the hair loss was psychological. They lost their hair because they believed chemotherapy caused hair loss. And there is more," Mary continued, allowing no lapse in the conversation. "In another group, 30 percent of the people got sick on their way to chemotherapy. They experienced nausea not after the drug had been administered, not during the administration, but before—in anticipation of chemotherapy.

"I realized my beliefs and attitudes contributed to the severity of my side effects. Of course that doesn't mean no one will never experience hair loss or mouth sores or be nauseous again. But it does mean that there is a psychological component to side effects, and we can work to control that component.

"In short, the belief we want to encourage is that the treatment is our friend. And as our friend, it is effective in helping overcome the physical aspects of the illness. It is fair to assume, then, that the side effects will, most likely, be very minimal."

"You're asking a lot," said the man. "I'm supposed to start radiation. And I don't see those burning rays as friends at all."

Mary continued, "The Cancer Conqueror taught me that I needed to believe in my treatment program even more than the physician who prescribed it did! That was a revelation to me. She went on to say that the treatment program was something I needed to get excited about. I would need to align myself with the treatment, believe in its effectiveness, and think of it as a welcome ally. I admit that I spent a lot of time nurturing this belief."

More notes. The man was starting to see something. The Cancer Conqueror was right. There was more to cancer than just the physical aspects.

"But even more important than beliefs about the disease, the treatment, and the side effects," continued Mary, "are the beliefs we have about our role in the cancer journey."

"What do you mean?" asked the man.

"Beliefs are fascinating," said Mary. "For me they started with the thought that my role would be that of the passive and submissive patient, sort of, 'Okay, Doc, whatever you think is best.' I thought I would just show up and receive treatments. I didn't think there was much else I could do.

"Then I was fortunate again. The same library where I found the facts on side effects had more information on other aspects of the cancer experience. Soon I was reading books on the role I could assume with my medical team, with the disease, with the treatments, and with my family. For the first time I was able to exercise some personal control over the illness. I was able to see my role as managing a total treatment program that included my medical team, my mind, and my spirit.

"I spent additional hours on the Internet where I studied and worked. I developed a fighting spirit. I fanned the flames of my will to live," said Mary with enthusiasm that was contagious. "If there was a book, I read it. If there was a tape, I listened to it. If there was a Web site, I visited it. Or a video, I watched it. I made notes and summaries of nearly everything on my type of cancer. There is no question in my mind that my self-education was a crucial part of the process of getting well. As it turned out, I had a vital role to play.

"Yet as helpful as all those things were, as important as the self-education process was, I always kept coming back to mind and spirit. It became apparent to me that mind and spirit were the key components of my treatment plan. They were also directly under my control. It led me to what I consider one of the single most powerful beliefs I had ever nurtured. I came to see that even though I had cancer, I was not cancer."

"Whatever do you mean?" asked the man.

Mary smiled as she explained. "I mean to say that by seeing myself not just as my body, which was riddled with cancer, but also as my mind and my spirit, which were very alive and ready to soar with energy, I was then able to make an important distinction. I was able to separate who I was as a person from what I had as a disease. I had control over my mind and spirit! And my mind and my spirit had cancer only if I allowed it.

"Who I was as a person was much more than what I had as a disease. That's what I mean when I say, 'Even though I have cancer, I am not cancer.' That is a mighty powerful belief."

❧❧❧

Even though I have cancer,
I am not cancer.

❧❧❧

The man caught up with his notes. "Tell me more," he said.

"The Cancer Conqueror taught me other beliefs," said Mary. "One of the most powerful was about the cancer cells themselves. Once I said to the Cancer Conqueror that it was terribly frightening to think of the cancer eating away inside my body. That's when she gently but forcefully corrected this false belief. I remember her words well: 'Cancer cells don't eat other cells. Cancer cells are weak and confused cells.' She went on to explain that the cells themselves are not intelligent. They don't make up a bodily organ. Instead, they have gone mad. They are confused."

"That's true," said the man. "I always believed that the cancer was all-powerful. That's a dangerous untruth, isn't it?"

"Yes," Mary confirmed. "It relates to another important belief that brings a new perspective to our treatment. Right in our own bodies is the mortal enemy of cancer cells, our very own immune system. You see, it is not that the surgeons, the radiation, or perhaps the chemotherapy and other treatments are so all-powerful. They themselves can't actually cure the cancer. No! The truth is that those treatments help the body's immune system heal itself—from within! The medical team plays a supporting role to the body's own healing power! Isn't that a revelation?"

The man sat contemplating what he had just heard. This was powerful, a totally different perspective than he had ever before believed. He realized the truth he was hearing could have a far-reaching impact on his own program for recovery. "Yes," he said, "I think I'm beginning to understand the significance of what you just said."

Mary went on. "The Cancer Conqueror taught me that cancer has significant psychological, emotional, and spiritual components. We can understand more about these aspects by looking at stress and the way we handle it. The important thing to realize is that mismanaged stress can lead to both a physical and a psychological reaction that primes the body to respond. This priming is a mental phenomenon. If we mentally respond by suppressing or over-expressing, we give the body confusing signals. The result is that our immune systems become compromised and less effective in warding off potential cancer cells.

"These essentials are documented in a growing field combining science and psychology called psychoneuro-immunology. It's a scientific discipline that recognizes mind and spirit do affect cellular biology. Thoughts of fear, anger, and guilt can lead to sickness on more levels than just the physical. Yet thoughts of love, joy, and peace lead to health and well-being."

The man put all this hopeful information in his notes. Most of what Mary said was new to him.

The man hesitated a moment. "Does this all mean that I gave myself cancer?"

"No, no!" said Mary. "That's much too rigid a view. You didn't give yourself cancer. However, the inability to handle stress constructively, to resolve conflicts creatively, and to manage anxieties effectively may have contributed to the beginning of illness. Of course, it wasn't a conscious decision. We never set out to give ourselves cancer. But yes, we may have contributed to the onset on a subconscious level.

"Now, here's the hopeful part. If you recognize that you may have contributed to your illness, then you must also believe that you have the power to contribute to your recovery. The psychological and spiritual components can work either for us or against us. The choice is ours."

The man nodded to indicate his thoughtful understanding. This belief was starting to make sense. And it was opening a door of hope.

"Perhaps understanding the context will help," Mary added. "Behind all these statements lies a revolutionary assumption that needs to be understood and believed at a deep level. The assumption is this—cancer is a process."

"I'm afraid you'll have to explain that a bit more," said the man.

"Conventional medical wisdom teaches us that cancer is a thing, a spatial entity or physical condition. My doctors talked about cancer as tumors. They talked about cancer as an abnormal state marked by those tumors. To them the word *cancer* was a noun—a thing."

"That is, of course, true," said the man.

"It is." Mary nodded. "But it is also a rather shallow definition of cancer. For example, I once thought of a golf ball as simply a round, white sphere with dimples in its surface. But that was before I saw a golf ball that had been sliced in half. There was the outer white, dimpled shell, all right. But there was also much more. Right under the surface was a deep red, rubberized coating. This covered and secured the next layer, which was made up of tan-colored rubber bands. They were tightly wound all around inside the ball. And in the very center was a hard, black rubber ball about the size of a large pea.

"Now for me to define a golf ball as round, white, and dimpled after seeing the cut-in-half ball would be incomplete. The same is true for cancer."

"I still don't understand what you're saying," said the man.

"Just this. Examine your own cancer experience beyond the obvious appearances. Open your mind to the full dimensions of the idea that cancer is more than a physical condition. Cancer is not a disease of which you are a victim. It is a process which you can master.

❧❧

Cancer is not a disease

of which you are a victim.

It is a process which you can master.

❧❧

"The medical community uses *cancer* as a noun. I encourage you to make *cancer* into a verb, an action verb! I challenge you to start to think, see, and feel yourself as 'cancering.'"

"Cancering?" asked the man.

"Yes," said Mary. "The verb *cancering* shifts our focus away from a disease we have and brings our attention to the process we are going through."

"Cancering," mused the man. "It has a strange sound to it."

"Good," said Mary. "That strange sound will help remind you that this is a process and that you have an important role."

"Will you trace this cancering process?" asked the man.

"Okay," said Mary, "let's walk through the typical steps.

"First, we need to understand that not every cancer patient's experience would fit this pattern. Certainly there are genetic causes of cancer. Some people are born with that unfortunate physical predisposition. And there is no question that carcinogens in our environment, in our foods, all around us, can trigger malignancy.

"Even so, there is increasing evidence that most cancers are lifestyle-related. In fact, the percentage may be much higher than scientists first imagined. Smoking, poor diet, excess weight, lack of exercise, all correlate with the onset of a wide range of cancers. What's more, one group of researchers found that more than 90 percent of their patients could trace the onset of cancer to a period of high stress. The researchers went so far as to say that, in their opinion, this same percentage probably applied to nearly all cancers."

"To stress? Astounding," said the man.

"The evidence is becoming overwhelming. Lifestyle is the key to preventing cancer as well as to reversing cancer. Our emotions are the pivotal issue. Many times the body will start cancering because of prolonged emotional conflict that has its roots in stress. And this emotional conflict—feelings of fear, hostility, guilt, grief, hopelessness, and despair—can lead to psychological depression. Today we have over thirty years of scientific evidence of a direct link between psychological depression and immune system depression. The result can be the onset of disease.

"Now, we need to make a careful distinction. This is not to say that all people who are having emotional distress will start cancering. It *is* to say that the cancering process is often triggered on the emotional level. Perhaps the first symptoms are barely detectable. And it may be months, even years, before physical symptoms occur. The physical symptoms eventually compel the patient to seek a medical diagnosis, and a treatment plan is then initiated. And while a proper treatment program on the physical level is mandatory, I encourage you to understand that the cancering process is far more inclusive. The physical portion—the tumor—is only a signpost in the process."

The man sat silently for a moment. "My intuition accepts this. But my rational mind wants to resist it."

Mary said, "Are you assuming that cancering excludes the conventional medical understanding? Cancering includes cell biology. We are simply opening our minds to go beyond the limits of that thinking. Because the truth is, cancering is both rational and intuitive. What we seek is a fully integrated approach—body, mind, and spirit.

"Believe it, cancer doesn't just happen to us. It can spring from inner disharmony, physical or emotional or spiritual. And this has two implications. One is responsibility. We may have been responsible, at least subconsciously, for contributing to the onset of the illness. But the second implication is opportunity. Cancer is a reversible disease, and there are patients who happily experience reversal every day. Our central task in recovery is to choose harmony at the level of mind and spirit. Only then can we help our bodies regenerate and achieve physical harmony. This is truly conquering cancer. And in conquering, we may even cure it."

Mary continued, "The Cancer Conqueror likes to help us reframe the meaning of cancer. By reframing, she means looking at the illness in a different light. This perspective includes new ways to consider several beliefs about the illness, the treatment, and our roles. But the Cancer Conqueror encourages us to accept the primary belief that cancer is a message to change.

⚜⚜

Cancer is a message

to change.

⚜⚜

"Yes, cancer certainly has a physical, cellular component. And yes, it can be life-threatening. But even though this is true, cancer is foremost a warning for us to change. The Cancer Conqueror calls this change *resolve*. When we resolve those areas in our lives where there is unrest, where there is anxiety, we make changes that will nurture love, joy, and peace. That's truly conquering cancer. The body will often respond physically to renewed feelings of hope. The mind's resolution of conflicts is often followed by the body's resolution of disease. This is true because body, mind, and spirit work together as one system.

"Our task, then, becomes one of identifying those areas that need resolution, fulfilling those needs, and choosing positive options for the future. Cancer becomes a message to change."

The man looked at all his notes. He wanted to spend time studying the implications of all this for himself.

"I know you need time to study," responded Mary. "Work this week on replacing negative beliefs with positive beliefs. I will arrange a meeting next week with one of the most beautiful people you will ever meet. Her name is Barbara, and she will teach you about resolving, one of the most important steps in conquering cancer."

Mary made the call; the time was set.

"Let me leave you with the Cancer Conqueror's favorite story about beliefs. One of her heroes is Christopher Columbus. At that point in history, everyone believed that the world was flat. But Columbus decided to challenge that belief. He took a chance, and the world has never been the same since! He was a real conqueror!

"Our beliefs about cancer are like that. You are a modern-day Columbus about to start a journey. Some people will tell you that there is no hope, that the world is flat. Don't believe it! Instead, start the journey. Choose to become a cancer conqueror!

"In a real sense, what you believe about this journey is what you'll experience. You will choose your beliefs. Make certain you do not accept hand-me-down beliefs that lead to despair. Make certain that your beliefs empower you, that they serve you well.

"Ask often, 'Do my beliefs instill despair or do they inspire hope?' You choose."

The man left, touched by Mary's power and authority. He was so impressed that he stopped his car down the block, got out his notebook, and right there made a summary of the positive beliefs.

❧ POSITIVE BELIEFS SUMMARY ❧

The Illness

1. I do not believe cancer is synonymous with death.
2. I believe cancer cells are weak and confused; they don't "eat" other cells.

The Treatment

3. I believe treatment is effective against these weak and confused cells.
4. I believe the side effects, if any, can be controlled.
5. I believe my own immune system overcomes cancer cells daily.

My Role

6. I believe I am personally responsible for my cancer journey.
7. I believe I manage my total treatment program.

8. I believe I can control the emotional, psychological, and spiritual aspects of my journey.
9. I believe I am "cancering." It is a process I can master.
10. I believe cancer is a message for me to change.

꙳ Readers' Choice ꙳

Our story continues on page 67. If you feel ready to begin exploring your belief system, consider the following exercises now. If you do not feel ready, you can continue with the story and return to these exercises later.

🦋 BELIEVE: 🦋
RECOVERING A SENSE OF THE POSSIBLE

Change your mind, change your health. That may be truer than we ever dared believe. Beliefs create actions. Actions create results. Results confirm beliefs. This is how self-fulfilling prophecies become reality.

Throughout the annals of cancer there are legions of people who, despite all odds, succeeded in achieving wellness. They found strength to carry them over, under, around, and through seemingly insurmountable obstacles. I believe the same is possible for you.

One of the chief barriers to attaining and accepting healing is the limits imposed by our beliefs. We have limited notions of what we can accomplish. Many times we believe that healing is not possible, that our personal case is fundamentally different, or that while others may be able to effect healing, we lack the inner resources or the moral goodness to attain wellness.

What follow are some suggestions for your thoughtful consideration. These are offered lovingly; I'm not demanding answers to any of these queries. I simply invite exploration of the set of beliefs you bring to the cancer recovery process.

Knowing that we all live somewhere between belief and disbelief, rate yourself openly and honestly. There are no right or wrong answers. Unless you choose to share, you are the only one who will see your responses. Thousands of fellow cancer survivors have found it highly empowering to explore the implications of the beliefs they hold. I predict you will benefit too.

Examine the Depth of Your Beliefs

Consider each statement. Indicate your level of belief by circling the relative value from 10 to 1, 10 indicating that you strongly believe, one that you strongly disbelieve. Reflect on your level of intensity surrounding each belief.

❧ Cancer is more than a physical illness.

Strongly believe		Somewhat believe		Not certain either way		Somewhat disbelieve		Strongly disbelieve	
10	9	8	7	6	5	4	3	2	1

Thought Starters: Do I believe that cancer is something more than cellular biology? What cultural and scientific beliefs does this challenge?

_____

_____

_____

✖ Cancer is not synonymous with my death.

Strongly believe		Somewhat believe		Not certain either way		Somewhat disbelieve		Strongly disbelieve	
10	9	8	7	6	5	4	3	2	1

Thought Starters: Is a belief like this empowering or actually self-deception? What benefits might result if I wholeheartedly embrace this belief? What if I reject it?

_____

_____

_____

_____

_____

_____

_____

_____

_____

_____

_____

❧ My cancer cells are weak and confused.

Strongly believe		Somewhat believe		Not certain either way		Somewhat disbelieve		Strongly disbelieve	
10	9	8	7	6	5	4	3	2	1

Thought Starters: What mental picture of cancer cells do I carry? What image might serve me best?

_____

_____

_____

_____

_____

_____

_____

_____

_____

_____

_____

_____

_____

_____

_____

❧ My treatment plan is highly effective.

Strongly believe		Somewhat believe		Not certain either way		Somewhat disbelieve		Strongly disbelieve	
10	9	8	7	6	5	4	3	2	1

Thought Starter: Do I understand how the actual therapy is intended to work? Does it seem scientifically plausible? Is it consistent with known principles? What is my confidence level in the practitioner and allied health care providers? Is the treatment delivered in an environment that is physically safe and emotionally nurturing?

❧ The side effects of my treatment are minor and can be largely controlled.

Strongly believe		Somewhat believe		Not certain either way		Somewhat disbelieve		Strongly disbelieve	
10	9	8	7	6	5	4	3	2	1

Thought Starter: What specifically do I fear most about potential side effects?

_____

_____

_____

_____

_____

_____

_____

_____

_____

_____

_____

_____

_____

_____

❧ My immune system has the potential to effectively control malignant cells.

Strongly believe		Somewhat believe		Not certain either way		Somewhat disbelieve		Strongly disbelieve	
10	9	8	7	6	5	4	3	2	1

Thought Starter: What could I do to further enhance my immune function?

_____

_____

_____

_____

_____

_____

_____

_____

_____

_____

_____

_____

_____

❧ I am in charge of my total treatment plan.

Strongly believe		Somewhat believe		Not certain either way		Somewhat disbelieve		Strongly disbelieve
10	9	8	7	6	5	4	3	2	1

Thought Starters: What elements, beyond medicine, can I add to enhance my total treatment plan? How can I remain in charge of this program?

_____

_____

_____

_____

_____

_____

_____

_____

_____

_____

_____

_____

_____

_____

_____

_____

❧ Emotional, psychological, and spiritual health is a choice.

Strongly believe		Somewhat believe		Not certain either way		Somewhat disbelieve		Strongly disbelieve	
10	9	8	7	6	5	4	3	2	1

Thought Starter: What can I do to choose wellness during times of doubt and fear?

❧ I am "cancering" as opposed to having cancer.

Strongly believe		Somewhat believe		Not certain either way		Somewhat disbelieve		Strongly disbelieve	
10	9	8	7	6	5	4	3	2	1

Thought Starters: How is this understanding different from the strictly biological definition of cancer? How does this understanding empower me?

Cancer is a message for me to change.

Strongly believe		Somewhat believe		Not certain either way		Somewhat disbelieve		Strongly disbelieve	
10	9	8	7	6	5	4	3	2	1

Thought Starters: Areas for change that might produce immediate benefits in my well-being include:

Diet_____

Exercise_____

Medical treatment_____

Emotional outlook _____

Relationships_____

Beliefs_____

Attitudes_____

Career_____

Purpose in life_____

Spiritual life _____

Other _____

For the Advanced Wellness Student

With a cancer diagnosis, feelings of hope and despair are in a constant tug-of-war. One day we may tune in the message of healing but the next day discount it as misguided or impossible. Wellness can be elusive. As soon as the situation looks desperate, we rule out what is possible before allowing the potential to unfold.

> *It amazes me how many cancer patients do not believe they can get well. Think of a bell-shaped curve; I have observed that at one end, 10 to 15 percent of patients actually welcome cancer and consider it an honorable way to die. In the middle of the curve, 70 to 80 percent of patients seem to just go along, dutifully fulfilling their passive role assigned by the doctor. At the far end of the curve is another 10 to 15 percent. These are the cancer conquerors. The most profound difference . . . is the set of underlying beliefs this group brings to the process.*
>
> —Greg Anderson,
> *1998 PBS television special,*
> Creating Incredible Wellness

Beliefs, and the resulting attitudes and expectations, constantly contribute to actual experience in all areas of life, including the experience of cancer. This much is clear: Beliefs can be chosen. But we seldom consciously choose them. Perhaps we have simply accepted beliefs for many years, like the conventional wisdom surrounding cancer. Perhaps we had beliefs imposed from parents, co-workers, or friends. We may have picked up other people's beliefs and made them our own. They may or may not be true or helpful.

Now I ask you to look deeply, deeper than ever before, and take a personal inventory that will heighten your awareness of your beliefs. Please respond in the open spirit of self-discovery.

❧ **One belief I have heard others espouse about cancer is**

_____

_____

_____

_____

_____

_____

_____

_____

_____

_____

_____

_____

❧ **My greatest fear about cancer is**

_____

_____

_____

_____

_____

_____

_____

_____

_____

_____

_____

_____

❧ **My fear of cancer stands in the way of my wellness by**

_____

_____

_____

_____

_____

_____

_____

_____

_____

_____

_____

_____

_____

Believe it or not, we can change our beliefs. We may habitually choose the same belief over and over: "I'm going to die of breast cancer just like my mother." "Oh God, ovarian cancer is so painful and frightening." "I may fight, but the cancer means my eventual demise." The fundamental belief is, cancer means death. It may not seem as if we are choosing the belief, but we did make the original choice.

❋ **What are three beliefs that would immediately help me begin to heal?**

_____

_____

_____

_____

_____

_____

_____

_____

_____

_____

_____

_____

_____

_____

❧ **What is one deeply held belief I would like to change? How can I best do that?**

_____

_____

_____

_____

_____

_____

_____

_____

_____

_____

_____

Beliefs can also be hidden and remain powerful guiding forces. If we are honest, we recognize there are moments when we are our own worst enemies. On the one hand, we take ourselves seriously and don't want to look like fools pursuing some false hope of recovery. On the other hand, we don't take ourselves—or God—seriously enough. Increasing our awareness of hidden beliefs increases our ability to respond positively.

❧ **I make myself sick by**

_____

_____

_____

_____

_____

_____

_____

_____

_____

_____

_____

_____

❧ **I become ill when I try to avoid**

_____

_____

_____

_____

_____

_____

_____

_____

_____

_____

_____

_____

_____

❈ **When I was sick as a child, my mother always**

_____

_____

_____

_____

_____

_____

_____

_____

_____

_____

_____

_____

❦ **Are any of these "hidden belief factors" adversely influencing your journey to wellness? If so, how does this new awareness direct you to respond?**

_____

_____

_____

_____

_____

_____

_____

_____

_____

_____

_____

Personal beliefs establish personal parameters. I ask you to believe in your vast potential for cancer recovery. I have seen it in my own life; I believe it is equally possible for you. Just because you now have cancer does not automatically mean you will have it a year from now. Cancer is a reversible disease. Believe it.

Are you aware of all your wellness assets? Awareness is the first step in deploying them. You and I are able to draw—

physically, emotionally, and spiritually—on an unlimited wellness account. We tend to draw very limited amounts compared with the resources available to us. This is the hour to tap into all your substantial reserves.

Today, vow to believe recovery is possible . . . for you . . . beginning now.

❧ Be Gentle ❧

Nurture yourself. After you complete these exercises, I suggest you take a break from your wellness work. Contemplate the important issues raised. Listen carefully to your inner wisdom; healing knocks softly. Return to the story after you have rested.

4

Cancer Conquerors Resolve

Early the following week, the man was at the door of Barbara's home. The first thing he noticed about Barbara was her smile. It was that same kind of joyful expression he had seen in Mary and in the Cancer Conqueror. And Barbara's voice, calm and soothing, was another indication of her obvious warmth. They made their way to the patio.

"How is your journey progressing?" Barbara began.

"Well, I've just started," replied the man. "But already the difference in my beliefs is significant. I'm less frightened of the disease. And I also feel more confidence in my treatment and in my medical team."

"Excellent," said Barbara. "And where are you in terms of your role?"

"My role is the area that confuses me most. Frankly, I

really wonder if what I think or feel will have much effect on the cancer. So I'm not sure about my role."

"Let's discuss that," said Barbara. "The Cancer Conqueror teaches us that much of our role is in the area she calls resolve. Resolve starts with some fundamentals—diet and exercise. Good nutrition is essential for recovery. Make a shift toward a plant-based, low-fat, low-salt, low-sugar diet. Consider nutritional supplements, including vitamins, minerals, and herbs. Guidelines on both are available from the Cancer Recovery Foundation of America. I encourage you to become your own nutrition expert. I want you to act on the belief that what you put in your body is very important. You deserve the best in nutrition, especially now. Tell me, does your diet meet those standards?"

"Well, I'm trying. Changing old habits isn't easy," said the man.

Barbara's silence spoke volumes. Finally she continued, "You don't have a habit to change so much as you have a decision to make. It's just like exercise. Most people have significant room for improvement here. Just know this—even patients with limiting physical conditions can maintain an exercise program. The type of exercise and the frequency is your decision. The benefits are both physical and psychological. The Cancer Conqueror personally established a half hour each day as her exercise goal. I did the same and chose walking. Similar to your nutrition research, study the literature available from the Cancer Recovery Foundation of America and become your own exercise expert. Remember, the goal here is to feel more energized, not to become an Olympic athlete."

Barbara paused. The man was silent. After a while she went on. "As important as nutrition and exercise are, when the Cancer Conqueror talks about resolve, she is actually putting the emphasis on issues of a psychological and emotional nature. In fact, she is really starting at the spiritual point of loving ourselves. Unless we have a healthy respect for ourselves, we probably won't eat right or exercise.

"Resolve asks us to look deep within to focus on identifying and clearing our lives of emotional roadblocks and self-destructive behavior. This is a critically important exercise because the resolve principle is based on the premise that emotions affect us physically."

"Is that really provable?" asked the man.

"I'm not certain what you require in terms of proof," continued Barbara. "The whole area of psychoneuro-immunology, or PNI for short, is documenting this mind-over-illness phenomenon. The evidence suggests it is very real. I encourage you to be open to the possibilities.

"Simply stated, the Cancer Conqueror urges us to acknowledge that beliefs, attitudes, and feelings go together to create a mental and emotional outlook toward life, an emotional lifestyle. Those emotions, either positive or negative, translate to the physical. Our beliefs, attitudes, and feelings lead to illness or wellness.

❦❦

Beliefs, attitudes, and feelings

lead to illness

or wellness.

❦❦

"Perhaps even more astounding, the Cancer Conqueror teaches us that emotions can play a central role in cancer's onset and course."

"Wait," interrupted the man. "You're saying things that aren't really proven. I'm a tough-minded businessman. I need proof. Anyway, I thought we were going to talk about resolving, not emotions."

Barbara was surprised at his resistance. How could she break through? Could his reaction be a clue to his message to change? While it wasn't Barbara's style to be confrontive, she heard herself firmly telling the man, "Please, listen carefully. Listen with your mind, don't just hear with your ears."

The man stared at her. It wasn't hard to sense his discomfort. Or was it thinly disguised contempt?

"We *are* talking about resolve," continued Barbara. "Emotions are the core issue of resolving. I am not a medical doctor or researcher. However, PNI experts have given us overwhelming evidence that emotions occupy a central role in health. Consider this: Cancer cells are regularly present in virtually all people. Yet relatively few of these people become ill. That's because the body's immune system is so powerful; it is the natural enemy of abnormal cells. The immune system routinely contains or destroys these cells, allowing them to be carried away through natural bodily processes.

"Yet, when a malignant cell is not destroyed, what is behind the immune system's less-than-optimal functioning? What lapse in the body's defenses might allow these cells to develop into a life-threatening malignancy? And why has it developed now? What may have caused the immune system to function at less than full capacity, when for years it operated so effectively?

"Some people answer this by insisting it is a matter of genetics. Others say diet. Still others teach that it is carcinogens in the environment. All these may make a contribution to answering the question Why cancer now? But none offers a full explanation."

Barbara leaned forward and touched the man's arm. "Listen very carefully," she said. "This is perhaps as close as I will get to offering you the proof you seem to need."

The man sat quietly. Barbara continued: "Genetics, carcinogens, and diet do play a role in the development of cancer. But why aren't they consistently the triggers? If there is a genetic predisposition to cancer, it has always been there. Diet may play a part, but in all likelihood the patient's diet has been rather predictable for years. And what about carcinogens? Most people have certainly been exposed to harmful substances before. So why now? What is different at this point in time that would allow the cancer to develop?

"It is at this point that PNI brings us back to the emotional components. What is different? Research is providing clear and convincing evidence that the development of cancer requires more than just the presence of abnormal cells. It also requires suppression of the body's natural defenses, the immune system. And the difference that could suppress the immune system? Changed emotional states."

The man was listening intently.

"Not only changed emotional states, but charged emotional states. Fear. Anger. Guilt. Hostility. All negative

emotional states. All commonly the results of mismanaged stress. All potentially capable of depressing the person and the immune system."

The man began writing notes again. Barbara glanced
down to see him underline the word *stress*.

"Much of the emotional aspect of cancer," she continued, "can be understood in the framework of stress.
Actually, the issue isn't the stress but how we respond to
stress."

"Tell me more," said the man.

"There are times when each of us faces highly stressful situations, when major emotional upsets seem to dom-
inate our lives. For decades science has documented that
illness is more likely to occur following highly stressful
events in people's lives. Some illnesses and their links to
stress—ulcers, high blood pressure, headaches, even some
heart disease—are readily accepted by the medical community. More recently, though, backaches, infections, and
even accidents have been seen to increase when a person
is chronically emotionally upset. What are your own
beliefs on this subject?"

"I believe it is true," agreed the man.

"It *is* true," Barbara went on. "And research is finding
more and more diseases that are linked to stress. Stress can
translate to changes in emotional states. Stress can challenge the way we relate to life. Perhaps it challenges our
habits, relationships, or our self-image. We 'feel' these
challenges emotionally."

"Isn't this like the 'fight or flight' response?" asked the
man.

"That's exactly it. The human body is endowed with
some fantastic capabilities that protect us. When our early

ancestors encountered a tiger in their path, there was an immediate reaction. Their breathing rate increased, muscles tensed, adrenaline charged their body, and their heart rate and blood pressure increased. When faced with a stressful situation, the body prepared the person either to stay and battle the tiger or to get away from the area as quickly as possible. Thus, the fight or flight response.

"Now, most of our planet's twentieth-century inhabitants don't normally have to deal with a wild animal in their path. But we do have to deal with mental tigers all the time. They are the stresses that can trigger the same bodily reactions.

"Instead of fighting or fleeing, which actually puts to use the adrenaline, the rapid heartbeat, and the faster breathing, today people often suppress or even deny their reactions to stress. The body's response to an emotional reaction does not get discharged. When we have no outward action available, the stress is internalized. And internalized stress can set us up for trouble.

"It's amazing. Research has found that stress is related to both negative and positive change. While an event like the death of a spouse ranks at the very top of the chart, and is certainly negative, a normally positive event, such as marriage, also produces significant stress. The point is change. Both the negative and positive events of life are often experienced as emotional conflict. It is not enough merely to analyze the stressful events or acquire new coping skills. Our point of power is to see beyond the stress and understand the emotions."

The man was quickly taking more notes.

"How do we manage the emotions associated with stress? Two things must happen in successful stress management. The Cancer Conqueror calls this management the Stress Solver System:

Change Your Perception of Yourself, and

Change Your Perception of Your Problem.

"It's that basic. We need to change our perception of ourselves and our ability to handle whatever life problems face us, particularly the stresses before cancer. Plus, we need to be able to perceive those problems as being less threatening. Arguably, you could solve the emotional conflict with just one change in perception. But increasing personal power and decreasing problem power is the essence of successful stress management."

More notes. Was she breaking through?

"The outcome of mismanaged stress is chronic emotional conflict. And continuing emotional conflict—chronic fear, anger, guilt, and hostility—leads to feelings of helplessness, hopelessness, and despair. From here, it is a short step to depression."

"Okay," said the man. "But this doesn't necessarily mean I'll get cancer."

"That's correct," said Barbara. "There is no 100 percent fixed link. But PNI studies are demonstrating there is a strong correlation between a depressed mind and a depressed immune system."

"How is that?" pursued the man.

"The heart of the immune system is the person's white blood cells. In a groundbreaking discovery, white blood cells were shown to have neuroreceptors. This means that feelings, our emotions, may be biochemically transmitted

to and 'felt' by the immune system. This is hugely significant. Just as negative and positive emotions can and do
affect the human spirit, they also seem to affect the immune
system. And a chronically depressed immune system can
lead to illnesses of many kinds, including cancer.

"Mind affecting body and emotions directing or even
controlling health makes perfect sense. Consider this.
When you have been ill, didn't it make you feel psycho-
logically down? In that case, body affected mind. It follows
that the reverse could also be true, that mind can affect
body. PNI is proving that even as we speak. This is much
more than theory."

The man looked thoughtful. "It fits my case," he said.
"I lost my job about a year ago. I've tried everything I can
think of, but there is nothing I can do to get suitable work.
It makes me feel so worthless. And I just hate my old boss.
I feel like such a failure."

Barbara now realized what the man's core issue was.
What he'd just said gave her the insight she needed to
assist him in unloading some of his emotional baggage.
Realizing that this was a delicate task of self-discovery, she
proceeded gently but firmly.

"Losing a job has to be difficult. It's unfair, and it affects
you and everyone around you. But let's stop for a moment
and apply what I've just said. Like it or not, losing a job
doesn't make you angry—you make you angry. Being
fired doesn't make you feel worthless—you make you feel
worthless. Nobody can label you a failure without your
permission. You choose those beliefs and attitudes. Feelings of helplessness and hopelessness were at the heart of
the development of my cancer. Let me share my experience, because in many ways it parallels yours.

"After thirty-two years of marriage and four wonderful children, my husband and I were divorced. I was consumed by self-pity. I described it by saying, 'He just left me.' I felt fearful, angry, and worthless. Then I became depressed. I viewed myself as a victim, a worthless failure."

"A victim under your husband's control, or just a victim out of control?" asked the man.

"Actually both," said Barbara. "And I even took it a step further. I saw myself as a victim of life. What I mean is that I let the crisis situation of the divorce touch all areas of my life. I suppose my reasoning was something like, If I am a failure as a wife and mother, I must be a failure at everything else. I have no value. Mentally and emotionally, I took everything to its worst possible conclusion.

"I then reasoned, But it's not my fault. It's my husband's fault. I am his victim. I am a victim of whatever life decides to serve me. My life is hopeless. I failed to realize hope and hopelessness are both choices. And I have a personal responsibility for those choices! Why not choose hope?

❧❧

Hope and hopelessness are both choices. Why not choose hope?

❧❧

"The Cancer Conqueror is currently helping a new friend who was recently diagnosed with prostate cancer. This man adopted a hopeless victim's stance that included a belief that cancer was a virtual death sentence. He also believed that he would become incontinent and impotent as a result of treatments. This man sees himself as being trapped by events beyond his control. He views himself as having no meaningful way to deal with these issues. He is filled with despair. He chose an emotional outlook that recognizes only helplessness. He's become a victim of circumstance. He has surrendered his power and personal accountability to choose hope. This is the classic victim stance."

"That's a very descriptive illustration," replied the man. "I can identify. The victim stance relates to my own situation of being out of work and developing cancer, doesn't it?"

"It might," said Barbara. "You be the judge of that." She was encouraged. The man was at least acknowledging the possible link between his emotional state and cancer. Barbara would carefully help him take the next step.

"For me," she continued, "the victim stance actually started with my self-image, including what other people thought I was supposed to do with my life. It is a typical pattern that the Cancer Conqueror describes like this:

1. A series of high-stress events tears at the person's self-image. I am faced with divorce. My self-talk, based on my self-image, says, 'I am supposed to be married.' Early in my life, I was taught marriage and motherhood meant success. People who get divorced are failures. Now that I am divorced, I am surely a first-rate failure.

2. The person's techniques for coping are inadequate in response to the self-image threat. My self-talk says, 'I am supposed to be a wife and mother. I

77

have no idea how a divorced person is supposed to function. I'm no longer in control.'

3. The person sees no way to resolve his or her emotional needs and becomes a victim. Self-talk speaks again. 'I can't go on. The situation is hopeless. I am helpless.'"

Barbara went on, "While my divorce is a rather obvious example, all of us adopt victim stances. A person in a dead-end job is afraid to move. An abused wife is fearful of leaving an abusive mate. Even attitudes like 'That's just the way I am' use the victim stance as a convenient way to avoid personal change and growth. But the fact is, we can choose to be victors instead of victims!"

❧❧

We can choose

to be victors

instead of victims!

❧❧

"This truly does relate to my being out of work," said the man. "I once viewed myself as being productive and successful. That became my self-image. That was me! When I was dismissed—I just hate the word *fired*—my whole reason for living ceased to exist. And I was defenseless. There was nothing I could do. I felt powerless. Life became unmanageable. And anger ruled to the point of rage. I was, and I guess I feel I still am, that victim. Nothing is within my control."

Wow, Barbara thought to herself, this could be a turning point! He has opened his mind to renewal.

The man's words came fast, with emotional force. Excellent! "I must break free from this victim's role."

Barbara spoke ever so sensitively. "You have just taken what is perhaps the most difficult step in conquering cancer. None of us wants to concede weakness or helplessness. But by doing so, you have opened yourself to untold possibilities. Once you free yourself from the role of victim, you can begin self-renewal. You can take on the role of victor."

The two sat silently for several moments.

"But what do I actually do?" continued the man. "I still feel so vulnerable. It's terrifying!"

Vulnerable didn't come close to describing how the man actually felt. He was emotionally naked. He had bared his soul to a virtual stranger. He didn't even talk to his wife about some of these feelings. It was frightening to be so open. He realized Barbara was answering his question, and he struggled to focus his mind on what she was saying.

"What you do now is begin to work on nurturing and renewing your mind and your emotions. The victim stance is full of toxic emotions. The victor stance is characterized by a calm and serene focus. Inner serenity is your first priority. That is the gateway to conquering cancer. A calm, quiet, focused mind and spirit is step one in the journey to wellness."

The man was reflective as he tried to understand some of the implications of what Barbara was telling him. "I'm not good at expressing my emotions," he admitted. "I have always believed that some feelings were best left unsaid. In fact, my father always said that people who talk about them seem pretty weak."

"Interesting that you should say that," said Barbara. "The Cancer Conqueror helped me so much when she shared the three most consistent traits of the cancer-prone personality:

"First, the typical cancer personality has a tendency to bottle up emotions. You've just shared your belief that feelings are best left unsaid. In my case I tended to play 'poor me' and go into a prolonged silence."

The man chuckled. "I've done my share of that."

"We all have," said Barbara. "This relates to the second tendency, excessive difficulty grieving loss. In my divorce, I felt as if I had been done the ultimate wrong. I felt abandoned by my husband. And when the children wouldn't take my side, I felt totally unappreciated. It was an overwhelming sense that I had lost everything I believed was important. And I continued living with those feelings until the Cancer Conqueror helped me begin to express my profound sense of grief over those losses."

The man responded, "I've never thought of my job loss in terms of grief. I suppose that is one framework in which to analyze it, though. I do know it has been a very difficult year. And I feel profoundly empty. I suppose some mourning might be called for."

Barbara nodded her agreement. The man was trying. He was working at this very sensitive assignment, and he was making progress. She continued: "The third common characteristic of a typical cancer profile is judgmentalism, being unduly critical of others. No question, I certainly did that, particularly where it concerned my husband. In fact,

I'm ashamed to say that I really went through life being critical of others. It was a twisted attempt to pull myself up by pushing others down."

The man was contemplative. "I suppose I carry some of all three of those personality traits."

"Perhaps," said Barbara. "Those personality characteristics can lead to emotional lifestyles dominated by fear, anger, hostility, and guilt. They can depress the immune system and allow cancer, and other illnesses, to flourish."

"Here we are again. I keep thinking I caused my own cancer!" The man sighed.

"No, now just recall our beliefs," said Barbara. "Remember that we probably did contribute to the illness on a subconscious level. But the key is this: If you acknowledge that you may have contributed to the illness, then by definition you must also acknowledge that you can contribute to your wellness."

"I do remember," said the man. "And I'm beginning to understand some of the ways I contributed negatively. Then it follows that I can change my lifestyle and contribute positively to my health and well-being."

"Exactly! Excellent!" said Barbara. "Remember, cancer is a reversible disease. You can contribute to that reversal."

❧❧

Cancer is a reversible disease.

❧❧

"That's powerful!" said the man.

He thought, This is simple yet so profound. On an intuitive level, the body-mind-spirit principles make sense. And if science can't fully explain something like electricity yet completely embraces it, why do I demand a full explanation of psychoneuroimmunology? I want to reverse my disease. I want life!

"Okay," said the man. "I want to get well! I'm choosing to live! Where do I start to resolve?"

Barbara beamed. *Choosing to live!* Those words affirming the will to live were powerful. Perhaps he had just turned the corner in his thinking.

"You've already started." She smiled. "What you do next is take a rigorous emotional inventory of yourself. The Cancer Conqueror gives us three questions that, if treated with respect, will lead us to higher self-awareness. You'll want to take notes here.

"First, ask yourself what high-stress, emotionally disruptive events happened to you in the year or two before diagnosis. This is the stress management issue. High-stress events can be identified in many patients. But what the Cancer Conqueror really wants us to do is get in touch with the way we reacted to those events. Did we respond to the events with paralyzing fear? Or did we get angry and let hostility turn to smoldering resentment? Or did guilt cause such a sense of shame that we may have felt we deserved some kind of punishment? And given the perspective of time, can we now look at different and more constructive ways of handling the situation?

"Second, what emotional needs might you be meeting or masking with the cancer?"

"What do you mean?" asked the man.

"Just this. Cancer partially fulfills many emotional needs. Cancer generates cards and get-well wishes from friends and relatives. It certainly has the power to allow you to be out of work; you can stay at home in bed and everyone will understand. Cancer elicits attention, no small amount of sympathy, and it may even serve as a means of obtaining nurturing from an otherwise nonnurturing spouse. Just think of cancer's power!

"Cancer is a great permission giver, allowing both patient and family an acceptable reason to say no to the demands of others. It can also provide a reason to say yes to things that have been put off or otherwise neglected in a person's life."

"I've never really thought about cancer that way before," said the man.

"The Cancer Conqueror," continued Barbara, "calls these cancer games. They are the secondary gains of the illness. Her real point is to look at the motivation behind our illness-related behavior. In our society, sickness is a powerful force, one that is often rewarded. Patients can manipulate this cultural belief, misappropriating it to meet their needs. Some people cling to cancer. It's their newfound way of fulfilling emotional needs that otherwise have gone unmet."

"That seems incredible to me," said the man.

"Incredible but true," said Barbara. "You will be invited to join a group of us who meet regularly. There you will meet a woman who not only has cancer but in her lifetime has had nine elective surgeries, currently takes eleven prescription medications, and claims this is the best she has felt in twenty-five years!

"She may be feeling better now than at any time in the

last twenty-five years, but the fact that she still recounts her many illnesses over and over again is a giveaway that she probably is receiving a great deal of fulfillment from her disease. It's her way of getting love and attention from her otherwise busy and emotionally distant husband.

"The Cancer Conqueror brings us back again and again to this point of examining what needs we might be meeting or masking with the illness. Why do I need this illness? and What am I gaining from cancer? become important matters to fully understand. So, spend time with these issues. Understand your own needs.

"This leads to the third question: What healthy options might you choose to fulfill these needs? Emotional needs are real. Denying them has probably been part of our problem. The Cancer Conqueror encourages us to recognize the real needs we feel; she encourages us to look at them squarely and not deny them. She also gives us permission to fulfill those needs but encourages us to do it in positive, healthy ways.

"So let's complete this issue of resolve. Here is an important point. I give you permission to give yourself permission to make certain your needs are met! What do you suppose is your number-one need?"

"Mine is simple. I need a job," said the man.

"Wait," said Barbara persuasively. "Look deeper. What are you really after?"

"What do you mean?" he asked. "I need work."

"Listen carefully. Let me offer some examples. In my case," continued Barbara, "I felt I needed to be married. Then the Cancer Conqueror helped me see that what I was really after was feeling secure, appreciated, and loved. But I was going about achieving those needs in a strange and self-destructive way. I was measuring the fulfillment of my needs by the amount of affection I received.

"When I did that, I always set myself up for disappointment; my husband and children could satisfy those needs only for short periods of time. And when I didn't receive attention and affection, I doubted my self-worth and began to fear rejection and abandonment. In my search for emotional fulfillment, I manipulated the people most dear to me. I think it caused them to resent me. In some ways, I can understand why my husband left, even after all those years we had together.

"The Cancer Conqueror helped me resolve nearly all those issues when she explained that our central task in resolving is to forgive—ourselves and others. Then she traced how certain processes help people release resentments and forgive both real and perceived wrongs, thus opening the mind and the body to healing. In fact, the Cancer Conqueror believes forgiveness is the most powerful psychospiritual component in getting well again.

❧❧

Our central task is to forgive—

ourselves and others.

❧❧

"Forgiveness was the breakthrough issue for me. It was the process of letting go of thoughts I harbored about people I perceived were harming me. It was equally a process of letting go of thoughts I had kept about harming others. I no longer saw myself as always being right and others as always being wrong. I was not always innocent and others always guilty. That thinking had put me into the blame game, where I always saw myself as a victim, not responsible for my own emotion well-being. I was surrendering power over myself to others. What a mistake! With forgiveness, I could choose differently. Now I could look upon myself and others with compassion, even love. In fact, for the first time I realized others were doing the best they could, given their level of awareness. And that applied to me as well. The issue was not blame at all.

"I remember one exercise that was most helpful. The Cancer Conqueror had us write a blame list. We wrote out individuals' names and next to the names what we blamed them for. Interestingly, the first name on the list had to be our own. Then, in a joyful ceremony, we crumpled our lists up in balls and threw them in a trash can. Then we took the trash can outside and burned the lists. It was marvelous! It's an event vividly etched in my memory. To this day, it helps me to stop blaming and start forgiving.

"Forgiveness became the major vehicle for me to use in the resolve process. I actively forgave others. I wished them well and imagined good things happening to them. It was truly a wonderful exercise that transformed my mind and spirit. And I forgave myself. I realized I could feel loved whether I was married or single, whether my children sided with me or my husband. I realized that my feeling loved was not dependent on others showing me attention or affection. It was instead dependent upon my showing love to others. Whenever I did, I felt loved. And I believe that by resolving this emotional conflict, I helped my body heal. Does that make sense? Does that fit you?" asked Barbara.

"I'm not certain," pondered the man.

"For me," Barbara continued slowly and deliberately, "the real need was to replace fear, anger, resentment, and guilt with love, joy, and peace. Being married and needing to feel loved were only symptoms of a deeper need. That may be true for you also.

"Time after time the people who conquer cancer are the ones who work systematically at resolving their emotional conflicts. The central issues are accepting personal responsibility on all levels of life, frankly examining fundamental beliefs, managing stress better, improving self-love, and nurturing better relationships through loving and forgiving. There's more, but that's the heart of it. I now understand that in order to conquer cancer a person needs to arrive at the point where he or she says, 'I value myself and I am unwilling to remain miserable. I will no longer live life this old destructive way.'"

The man was thoughtful as he finished his notes: ". . . unwilling to remain miserable . . . a new person."

"Your experience of extended unemployment is common. I'm thinking of a man who is part of our Cancer Conqueror support group who was also fired from his job. He was a senior officer in one of the largest companies in this city. In fact, his departure was carried in the newspaper. He felt disgraced. His entire self-image was centered on his job. And within one year, prostate cancer.

"He spent time with the Cancer Conqueror, who helped him analyze his deep resentment. 'I'm so mad because I don't have a job,' he said. The Cancer Conqueror helped him realize a new truth—perhaps he didn't have a job because he was so angry and hostile. He had to grasp his real need. For years he had harbored resentment. It was time to change—not just jobs but some very deep emotions."

The man listened intently as Barbara continued.

"It's rigorous work dealing with these emotions. They are at the heart of where we live every day. Just remember that our emotions don't just happen to us, we choose them."

❦❦❦

Our emotions

don't just happen to us,

we choose them.

❦❦❦

"That's an odd thought," said the man.

"At first it may seem odd, but examine it. As I shared, when my husband and I went through the divorce, I was the classic victim. Then cancer. The illness merely reinforced my victim stance. I became a servant of my fears, angers, and guilts. I chose negative emotions.

"It wasn't until the Cancer Conqueror helped me reframe these negative emotions and taught me forgiveness that I was able to realize I could actually determine my own emotions. I realized I need not be a captive of my toxic fear, anger, and guilt. Instead, I was, or at least could choose to be, a person of love, joy, and peace.

"For the first time, I realized that we can't control life but we can control our response to life. And I began to understand cancer as a message—as negative feedback—that up to now I had not been making the best choices. I changed. I chose life. I chose to *live!*"

The man was silent, deep in thought.

Barbara paused for a moment, and when the man was ready, she continued. "It all brings us back to the core of resolve—the changing of our emotional lifestyles. By doing so, we prepare the body to heal. Clearing our lives of emotional turmoil is a *live* message. This is resolving!"

"It's interesting," said the man. "Resolve isn't changing the circumstances so much as changing ourselves."

"Precisely," said Barbara. "We can't change anyone but ourselves. That is the key. It's true. I became a cancer conqueror not because I went into remission. I became a cancer conqueror because I chose to become a new person!"

❧❧❧

You become a cancer conqueror

not because you go into remission.

You become a cancer conqueror

because you choose to become

a new person!

❧❧❧

Another pause. More reflection. "It all sounds so easy," said the man.

Barbara smiled. "Nobody will tell you it is easy. Simple? Yes. Easy? No. Just try to remember that change, like our emotions, is a choice. New choices are not easy. Pain is inevitable, but suffering is optional."

"Oh, that's good," said the man. "That's an excellent perspective. But how do I actually initiate all this? How do I make these changes real for me?"

Barbara reached for a piece of paper and began writing. "Here is the name and telephone number of a fellow journeyer. John has a whole new and exciting message for you to consider. And it is all centered on how to make these concepts work in your life. Call him and set up an appointment after you have begun to work through some of the resolve principles."

"I will," promised the man. "But before we quit today, will you help me summarize the principles we covered under resolve?"

"Of course," said Barbara. "Let's make a list."

Resolve Summary

1. Emotions affect us physically.
2. Beliefs, attitudes, and feelings lead to illness or wellness.
3. Fear, anger, and guilt can depress the immune system.
4. The Stress Solver System: Increase my personal power and decrease my problem power.
5. Hope and hopelessness are both choices. I can choose hope.
6. Instead of a victim, I choose to be a victor.

7. Cancer is a reversible disease.
8. My job is to forgive—myself and others.
9. Our emotions don't just happen to us, we choose them.
10. I become a cancer conqueror not because I go into remission. I become a cancer conqueror because I choose to become a new person!

❧ Readers' Choice ❧

Our story continues on page 117. If you feel ready to begin resolving some of your emotional issues, consider the following exercises now. If you do not feel ready, you can continue with the story and return to these exercises later.

❧ *RESOLVE:* ❧
LETTING GO OF FEAR, ANGER, AND GUILT

Most of us carry around a lot of emotional baggage. The contents are mainly variations of fear, anger, and guilt. This load is unnecessary and may even have contributed to the onset of cancer. The good news: Unburdening ourselves often contributes to healing.

The link between emotions and health is rapidly gaining a significant foundation of scientific proof. Dr. Yujiro Ikemi and colleagues in Kyoto, Japan, conducted a retrospective study of long-term survivors from cancers usually considered terminal. Why did they live? The patients all reported the onset of the disease during a time of severe "existential crisis." They then used the diagnosis of cancer as an opportunity to resolve the issues that led up to the disease. Finally, the patients committed themselves to carrying out God's will in their lives.

Dr. Steven Greer at King's College Hospital in England compared a group of women treated with mastectomy for breast cancer. Survival was nearly three times greater among those who developed a fighting spirit in response to the diagnosis compared with those who felt hopeless and helpless.

More recent psychosocial studies of cancer patients here in the United States confirm these findings. Dr. David Spiegel at Stanford University directed a study of breast cancer patients who participated in emotionally expressive groups. The findings: Participants lived twice as long as nonparticipants.

At UCLA, Dr. Fawzy Fawzy followed malignant melanoma patients who participated in emotionally supportive groups. Participants in a six-week program that taught better emotional coping skills lived twice as long as those in control groups who did not take part.

Your appreciation of the link between emotions and health is second in importance only to your understanding of the entire range of choices in physical treatments. The following exercises focus on increasing emotional awareness and defining optimal emotional choices. As the word *optimal* implies, perfect emotional awareness and the ideal emotional response are eternally unattainable goals; even the best of us fall short some of the time. Yet there remains a healthy emotional direction that holds out the very real hope of healing. These queries point you in that direction.

Tune Up Your Emotional Guidance System

Consider each statement. Indicate your level of belief by circling the relative value from 10 to 1. Reflect on your level of intensity—always, often, sometimes, seldom, never—surrounding each belief.

❧ I live with a vital awareness that my emotions play a major role in determining my health.

Always		Often		Sometimes		Seldom		Never
10	9	8	7	6	5	4	3	2	1

Thought Starters: How compelling do I consider the current scientific evidence regarding the mind-body connection? If I accept this concept, what are the implications concerning my current state of health?

_____

_____

_____

_____

_____

_____

_____

_____

_____

_____

_____

_____

_____

_____

_____

_____

_____

_____

❧ **I am aware of and can identify my emotions.**

Always		Often		Sometimes		Seldom		Never	
10	9	8	7	6	5	4	3	2	1

Thought Starters: List three people or circumstances that nearly always elicit fearful emotions from you. List three that elicit anger. And three that produce feelings of guilt. What thoughts typically precede each of these emotional responses?

_____

_____

_____

_____

_____

_____

_____

_____

_____

_____

_____

_____

_____

_____

_____

❧ **Once aware of my emotions, I am typically able to ask, "Does this warrant my becoming fearful (angry/guilty)?"**

Always	Often	Sometimes	Seldom	Never
10	9	8	7	6	5	4	3	2	1

Thought Starter: List a favorite response, such as, "Oh well, it's only my emotions," that could counter your negative responses to emotionally charged people and circumstances.

_____

_____

_____

_____

_____

_____

_____

_____

_____

_____

_____

_____

_____

_____

_____

_____

❧ I control emotions that are aimed at affixing blame on others or myself.

Always		Often		Sometimes		Seldom		Never	
10	9	8	7	6	5	4	3	2	1

Thought Starter: Identify the people or circumstances to whom you have attached blame for your emotional upsets. Write the people's names and/or the circumstances here.

_____

_____

_____

_____

_____

_____

_____

_____

_____

_____

_____

_____

_____

_____

✣ **I am appropriately assertive, making my needs known at the right time and in the right manner.**

Always		Often		Sometimes		Seldom		Never	
10	9	8	7	6	5	4	3	2	1

Thought Starter: List three things to which you recently should have said no. List three recent events in which you were overly assertive. What has been their toll on your health?

_____

_____

_____

_____

_____

_____

_____

_____

_____

_____

_____

_____

_____

_____

_____

_____

❧ **I carefully listen to others—and to myself—and am able to discern motives and intention.**

Always		Often		Sometimes		Seldom		Never	
10	9	8	7	6	5	4	3	2	1

Thought Starter: Describe a recent circumstance in which you listened with great care and were able to clearly understand the *why* behind the actions and events. How do you sense this was of emotional benefit to you?

_____

_____

_____

_____

_____

_____

_____

_____

_____

_____

_____

_____

_____

_____

❧ I am able to practice the healthful art of "release."

Always	Often	Sometimes	Seldom	Never
10 9	8 7	6 5	4 3	2 1

Thought Starter: List three people or circumstances and the corresponding emotions that you need to learn to let go of.

_____

_____

_____

_____
_____
_____
_____
_____
_____
_____
_____
_____
_____

❧ **I value myself and refuse to suffer through either despair or denial as I travel the cancer journey.**

Always		Often		Sometimes		Seldom		Never	
10	9	8	7	6	5	4	3	2	1

Thought Starter: List three personal actions you have found helpful in replacing emotions of fear, anger, and guilt with happiness, joy, and personal peace.

_____
_____
_____
_____
_____

_____

_____

_____

_____

_____

_____

_____

_____

I recognize cancer is, among other things, demanding of me a different emotional lifestyle.

Always		Often		Sometimes		Seldom		Never	
10	9	8	7	6	5	4	3	2	1

Thought Starters: From an emotional perspective, what are you gaining from this illness? Describe one example of how this illness is giving you permission to meet an emotional need for love, acceptance, or control. How might that need be better fulfilled? What changes will that require?

_____

_____

_____

_____

_____

_____

_____

_____

_____

_____

_____

_____

_____

For the Advanced Wellness Student

The first step in resolving conflict is an inward one; we must notice the typical emotional road maps by which we navigate. Awareness starts the process. If you completed the preceding exercises, you now have a keener insight into your emotional patterns. But there are subtler emotional lifestyle issues that are part of the experience of cancer. They relate to the ways cancer can actually benefit us.

At first glance, most people are surprised that having cancer carries any benefits at all. It does. Cancer most often changes the way people relate to one another. Many patients and support people develop new, usually more spiritual, perspectives on life. And cancer is often the catalyst to filling some unmet emotional needs. These side benefits can be positive and most meaningful. Hundreds of patients have told me, "I know this sounds strange, but I am actually thankful I went through the cancer experience." For these people, life takes on a new quality. Cancer has helped them live fuller and richer lives.

Some secondary gains, though, have a darker side. Cancer can become insidious and serve as a powerful lever to manipulate and control others. Our culture sanctions this because life-threatening illness is a powerful cultural force. Throughout virtually all societies, people who become sick are likely to receive certain automatic benefits. We tend to treat them better than people who are healthy. Certainly when people are ill they need treatment and nourishment—physically, emotionally, and spiritually. And it is wonderful when people receive it.

But many people feel as if they must become ill or stay ill in order to receive love and attention. In effect, we reward the ill and punish or withhold rewards from the well. Much is expected from those who are healthy; expectations are lowered for those with life-threatening illness. It's a widely accepted cultural norm.

To the extent that cancer is a means of fulfilling emotional needs, it tends to be critically important to many patients. People cling to and protect what is important. We say, "Oh no, surely that's not me." Let's be certain.

❧ **The relationship that has changed most from my experience with cancer is**

_____

_____

_____

_____

_____

_____

_____

_____

_____

_____

_____

_____

_____

❦ **This relationship has changed in the following ways**

_____

_____

_____

_____

_____

_____

_____

_____

_____

_____

_____

_____

_____

_____

❦ **Other relationships, responsibilities, and expectations that have changed as a result of my cancer include**

_____

_____

_____

_____

_____

_____

_____

_____

_____

_____

_____

Cancer comes bearing gifts. It is important to recognize those positive secondary gains so that the patient, the entire family, and the surrounding social support group can continue to help implement them. The goal is to incorporate the benefits into daily life and, after health is regained, keep them as more positive ways of meeting emotional needs.

It will benefit you to increase your awareness of the positive gains that cancer has demonstrated in your life. Complete the following prompts:

❧ **Cancer gave me the gift of permission to express my feelings and ask for my needs to be met in these areas**

_____

_____

_____

_____

_____

_____

_____

_____

_____

_____

_____

_____

❧ **Cancer gave me the gift of not taking the following for granted**

_____

_____

_____

_____

_____

_____

_____

_____

_____

_____

_____

_____

_____

_____

❧ **Cancer gave me the gift to stop postponing**

_____

_____

_____

_____

_____

_____

_____

_____

_____

_____

_____

_____

_____

❦ **Cancer gave me the gift of being able to say no to**

_____

_____

_____

_____

_____

_____

_____

_____

_____

_____

_____

_____

_____

_____

❧ **Cancer gave me the gift of not basing my life on what other people may think of me in the following areas**

_____
_____
_____
_____
_____
_____
_____
_____
_____
_____
_____

❧ **Cancer gave me other gifts that include**

_____
_____
_____
_____
_____

_____

_____

_____

_____

_____

_____

_____

_____

Now the challenge is to maintain the positive gains and without using cancer as a manipulative tool. Our emotional need for love and compassion is legitimate. Improving the quality of life, for ourselves and others, is an appropriate priority. Personal growth is a worthy pursuit. Cancer, and the transformation it calls us to make, can be the gateway to all this and more.

Perhaps it is time to consider some future strategies on living and how to maintain the real gains of cancer. Ask yourself these questions:

❧ **How can I continue to communicate more authentically than I did before I learned about my cancer diagnosis?**

_____

_____

_____

_____

_____

_____

_____

_____

_____

_____

_____

_____

❦ **How can I nurture this sense of team that my family and support network have developed?**

_____

_____

_____

_____

_____

_____

_____

_____

_____

_____

_____

_____

❧ **How can I allow more autonomy for myself and permit more autonomy for my family and loved ones?**

_____

_____

_____

_____

_____

_____

_____

_____

_____

_____

_____

_____

❧ **What must I do to maintain the internal permissions cancer gave me without clinging to the disease?**

_____

_____

_____

_____

_____

_____

_____

_____

_____

_____

_____

_____

❧ **When I think of being well again, what do I imagine will change?**

_____

_____

_____

_____

_____

_____

_____

_____

_____

_____

_____

_____

❧ When I think of being well again, do I imagine I will once again fulfill my responsibilities with similar intensity and at such breakneck speed? How will life be different?

_____

_____

_____

_____

_____

_____

_____

_____

_____

_____

_____

❧ When I think of being well again, will I still feel subject to the same pressures at work and at home? How will life be different?

_____

_____

_____

_____

_____

_____

_____

_____

_____

_____

_____

_____

_____

_____

_____

❧ **When I think of being well again, will I still be able to say no when I feel like it?**

_____

_____

_____

_____

_____

_____

_____

_____

_____

_____

_____

_____

Your emotional lifestyle is central to your recovery from cancer. You and I have the ability to choose our emotions, every day, in every situation. In the past we have allowed emotions to be chosen for us, accepting what came without regard for our well-being. Most times this strategy did not serve us well.

Today, vow to choose your emotional lifestyle. It is a critical lesson on the journey to wellness.

❧ Be Gentle ❧

Nurture yourself. After you complete these exercises, I suggest you take a break from your wellness work. Contemplate the important issues raised. Listen carefully to your inner wisdom; healing knocks softly. Return to the story after you have rested.

❧ 5 ❧

Cancer
Conquerors Live

The man spent an uncomfortable week trying to deal with the issues of resolve. It was no easy task. He did not fully appreciate being confronted with his own emotional conflicts. *It's forcing me to get in touch with some heavy issues. Aren't these things best left buried?* he thought. This was difficult, even frightening work. Yet he understood the connection between emotional and physical well-being. *I will continue resolving—gently,* he vowed.

The man made a lunch appointment with John to talk about *live*. Perhaps this would be an easier assignment. Maybe John would be able to help him through the difficult process of changing. He arrived at John's office early. The receptionist pointed to an open double door and said, "You'll find him in there. Go right in."

As the man entered, he saw John not behind his desk

but standing in front of it juggling three bright orange balls. "Come in," said John as soon as he saw the man. "Let's see how long I can keep these going!" John's personality immediately drew a stranger in. Along with it came a big, easy smile and an unassuming manner. Yet his clothes, his grooming, and his posture also commanded a certain respect for this unusual businessman. Here was someone you liked and wanted to know more about.

"Oops!" John laughed as one of the balls dropped to the floor. "I'm going to practice more tomorrow! Hello! Welcome!" He smiled as they shook hands. John's deep voice was melodious. "I've had some fruit brought in for us," he said as he gestured to the conference table. "Let's just eat our lunch right here. Make yourself at home."

After only a few minutes of pleasantries, John said, "You impress me as a person of high intelligence. And because of that, I am going to take a chance. I'm first going to tell you a story that I believe will help you always to recall the central point of *live*."

"Okay"—the man chuckled—"go ahead." You just had to like John. He was like a big teddy bear. And his directness was refreshing. Besides, how could you fault somebody who had already noticed your intelligence— someone who must be a keen observer of human talent? No doubt about it, John was joyful. He smiled as again he began his story.

"Once upon a time there was a handsome prince. On a walk in the forest, he met a wicked witch who was very evil. She waved her magic wand and turned the handsome prince into a frog. As the wicked witch was leaving the forest, she said, 'The only way this spell can be broken is with a kiss from a beautiful fair maiden.'"

John continued, the big smile widening across his face. It was obvious, he was having fun! "One day a beautiful fair maiden came to the edge of the pond where the prince-disguised-as-frog lived. Seeing his chance, he spoke to the maiden, telling her of his plight. 'And as the wicked witch left,' he concluded, 'she told me that the only way the spell could be broken would be by a kiss from a beautiful fair maiden. Will you kiss me and turn me back into a prince?'

"The princess looked at him. Certainly she didn't feel like kissing a frog. How could she really know if he was telling the truth? No, this was preposterous. Who had ever heard of a prince disguised as a frog? And even if there should be a prince under there, why was she the one who had to give the kiss? It was a lot safer not to get involved.

"But then the princess began to consider the situation more carefully—what if there really was a handsome prince under all that ugly green skin? What if he really was telling the truth? Just because she had never encountered this before did not mean it wasn't possible. And why shouldn't she be the deliverer of the kiss? It might actually be exciting to be involved, a whole new adventure."

John laughed as he went on. "What did she do? She took a chance! She trusted her positive instincts. She kissed that frog, and the handsome prince appeared. And they lived happily ever after." John smiled. "Now"—he chuckled—"I go through that whole story for this one reason. And that is so you will remember that our job is to become frog kissers!"

John leaned back and grinned. The man had to smile, too.

"A frog kisser? What does that mean?"

"What do you think it means?" asked John.

"I haven't the slightest idea," replied the man candidly.

John looked at the man. "Frog kissing. What we are talking about, my friend, is love—unconditional love. And the truth is, that kind of love conquers cancer!"

❧❧❧

Unconditional love

conquers cancer.

❧❧❧

"Love?" asked the man. "Is that where the journey leads?"

"It certainly does," said John.

"Tell me more," said the man.

"If I could give you just one insight on how to conquer cancer," said John, "it would be to love, to be a frog kisser. And my advice would be to love yourself first—to kiss the frog in the mirror.

"The Cancer Conqueror teaches that many people, particularly many cancer patients, grow up with the idea they are somehow flawed and their lack of perfection makes them unacceptable. People who feel like this often act as if they must cover up this central defect if they are to be accepted, if they are to have any chance for love.

"Feeling unloved and feeling as if they are not worthy of love, these people retreat into isolation and loneliness. This retreat is a natural outcome of hiding their fear that another person will discover the inner deficiency that makes them feel so unworthy.

"The Cancer Conqueror cites how often cancer patients tend to be perfectionist, overachieving workaholics who repress their real feelings in their busywork. They judge their worth by their work—how well they did it, how much of it they did, and how long they worked at it. And, even when successful, these people often don't feel good about their accomplishments. They may even resent others for not noticing their work."

The man raised his hand to stop John. "You're describing me, a perfectionistic, overachieving workaholic! And you're right, nobody ever appreciates what I've done!"

"There are some very heavy prices for living life by those standards," said John. "It's back to that whole thought of a central defect again. These people want to be judged by what they do—their work—rather than by who they are as individuals. And the trouble is, their good work is never good enough. And the praise, from self and others, is never quite loud enough!"

"Oh wow!" exclaimed the man. "That's me."

"Does this behavior often lead you to feelings of emptiness and disappointment?" asked John.

"Constantly." The man nodded.

"Because of their profound inner emptiness and their despair, people with this characteristic often come to view all their relationships in terms of finding something to fill the void. This is the conditional love you hear so much about. These people give love, give of themselves, give anything, only on the condition that they get something in return for it."

"Like what?" asked the man.

"It could be anything. People's conditions for love are vastly different. Some people want economic security. Some seek fame or power. Others want love and nurturing in return. Most seek approval from others; validation is what psychologists call it. The trouble with behavior that places conditions on love is that it is manipulative. It is conditional, contingent upon getting something back. It is an 'if love.' It leads to an even deeper sense of emptiness because it will always fail to satisfy."

"If the conditions were being met, it wouldn't fail. It would work just fine," contended the man.

"Not for long," insisted John. "We're talking about human beings, people with expectations that escalate. It is just a matter of time before either the expectations are not met or the people trying to fulfill those expectations come to see themselves as being manipulated and quit. But that's only the first level.

"On a deeper level, this 'if love' prevents the person from understanding his or her true and unique self. If you are always spending energy determining the degree to which your expectations are being met, and the degree to which you will return love, you'll never be able to understand the true you. The ego is always seeking fulfillment; the true self is never revealed. It is a vicious circle that results in perpetual disappointment, deepening emptiness, and personal despair. All are precursors of illness."

"Are you saying that I love conditionally?" asked the man.

"Yes. I do, you do, we all do," answered John. "At times in our life, we all love with *ifs*. The trouble is, it doesn't stop there. That despair born of loneliness often leads to something even more insidious—judgmentalism.

"This is the stage where people are constantly critical of people and circumstances that are different from their own views. The Cancer Conqueror points out that many people were brought up with a lot of *shoulds*, *oughts*, and *have to*s: A woman *should* be at home. A man *ought* to be a good provider. Children *have to* eat all their dinner. There are literally hundreds of these little rules.

"It's a miserable existence. Everything gets judged. Everyone is labeled as flawed and no good. All this is a subversive attempt by the judgmental person to build himself up while tearing others down. The vicious circle—disappointment, emptiness, and despair—continues."

"This is really depressing," said the man. "I thought we were going to talk about *live*."

John smiled. "We are, my friend. We're going to talk about how conquering cancer requires us to live, laugh, and love. But to do that, we need this perspective on judgmental and conditional love. The Cancer Conqueror once traced how crucial unconditional love really is. She believes that all disease has a lack of love at its roots. She explains how love that is judgmental and conditional leads to depression and thus allows physical vulnerability. Can you grasp her point? She even goes so far as to say that she feels all healing has at its roots the ability to give and receive unconditional love."

❦

Healing has at its roots

the ability to give

and receive

unconditional love.

❦

"I don't understand. What does this mean?" asked the man.

"Just think of live, laugh, and love. First we must live, we must appreciate the power of health's intangibles, especially the beliefs and attitudes that are rooted in hope. This is a very real hope that we can live positively here and now, even with cancer.

"And laugh, to mobilize humor, to help maintain the perspective that life still holds great joy.

"And love. It means that our task becomes learning to give and receive unconditional love. It means to stop judging.

"Live. Laugh. Love. That is our new aim."

The man was enchanted. Live, laugh, love. Could this actually be the guiding philosophy and strategy to his wellness? John was continuing. "The Cancer Conqueror puts this in clear perspective when she talks about three valid standards by which to judge. She feels there are moral standards, legal standards, and law-of-nature standards. Perhaps an example will help. Let's say friends with whom you have an appointment are late. Your initial concern for their safety soon turns to anger. 'They don't respect my time. They are always late. They make me mad. They're really inconsiderate people.' There's lots of judging going on here.

"But there is another choice. We could reevaluate our thoughts about the lateness in light of the three standards. Does their lateness break any moral law? Is this in the same class as murdering someone or intentionally harming another person? Does their lateness break any legal standard? Is this behavior in the same class as speeding at a hundred miles per hour? And does the friends' lateness go against any natural law? Is the behavior in the same category as chlorofluorocarbons damaging the ozone?"

"Okay." The man chuckled. "Those are pretty exaggerated examples."

"Not really. Those are just the types of thoughts that trigger judging all the time. The point is, if someone's behavior doesn't break a moral, legal, or natural law, forget it! Don't judge it! If we can just release ourselves from judgmental behavior, we are then free to live, laugh, and love. When we make positive, joyful, unconditional love—living, laughing, loving—our aim, it forms a powerful basis for health and healing.

"I am convinced that the energy we put into judging can be redirected to help us get well. In that sense, unconditional love is a powerful stimulant to our natural immune systems. Love is not merely emotional. It is physiological. In a real sense, love can always conquer cancer and often cures it too!"

John stopped as the man finished his notes. "It all relates to another facet of frog kissing, acceptance versus approval. It's the difference between accepting people for who they are versus approving of them for what they do, their behavior. This applies not only to how you relate to others but especially to how you see yourself.

"For example, you now know you are much more than your behavior; you have great worth outside your behavior. You have worth as a person, as a living human being in addition to what you may do, even in spite of what you may do! The key is to learn to truly accept your worth as a person even though you may not approve of your behavior."

The man was silent, deep in thought. Finally, in a whisper, he said, "Tell me more."

"Okay," said John, "let's go from looking within to looking without. Let's examine other people. They are just the same as you and me. Their worth isn't dependent upon what they do. We can decide to accept others as fellow citizens of the world, even though we may not approve of their behavior. Our task is to accept others, not approve of others."

❧❧

Our task is to accept others,

not approve of others.

❧❧

"Accepting and not approving removes me from having to be the judge, doesn't it?" asked the man.

"That's it," John agreed enthusiastically. "That's precisely it. It's so fundamental to well-being. You see, when we judge, we don't really see the other person, or ourselves, as whole. Most of us were brought up in an environment where the emphasis was on supposedly constructive criticism. This is usually a disguise for faultfinding. When we judge, we find fault and almost invariably label that person, or ourselves, as unworthy. We assume the other person to be wholly bad. We assume ourselves to be wholly unworthy.

"But if we can simply separate people from their behavior, we then find much to lovingly accept and celebrate. We go from being faultfinders to becoming lovefinders! Only then can we hear that strong inner voice saying, 'I love you and accept you just as you are.'"

The man was again silent. This was different . . . and, again, somewhat frightening. He thought he detected a fatal flaw in John's approach. If you decided to love, you left yourself vulnerable. "Other people will take advantage of that kind of love," said the man, voicing his doubts.

"Only if you carry expectations about receiving love from those people," said John. "People's reactions make little difference. It's what is coming from you, not what is coming to you, that makes the crucial difference."

The man contemplated all he was hearing. This was an entirely new way to see oneself and others. It meant assuming another new role.

John continued, "Perhaps the classic example is the case of the diners who go into a fashionable restaurant. They find the service deplorable and the waitress unfriendly and rude. Feeling angry and mistreated, the diners believe they are justified in their grievance and hostility and leave the waitress no tip. Now let's replay the scene from the start. This time let's assume that the patrons discover, just as they sit down, that the husband of the waitress died two days ago and she has five children at home who are solely dependent on her support.

"This changes everything. The customers adopt a new role that overlooks the behavior as threatening and sees the waitress as fearful, recognizing that she is calling out for love and acceptance. Their response accepts her as a person without having to approve of her actions and behavior. Their attitude is now loving, a response they demonstrate by leaving an extra large tip.

"Understand the difference," said John. "The scene was the same in each case. The characters were the same. The place was the same. The words were the same. However, in the first scene, the events were seen through the window of approval, with conditional love. And in the second, they were seen through the window of acceptance, of unconditional love. What changed was the patrons' role. Nothing else. They went from faultfinding to lovefinding. We can live life this very same way! We can conquer cancer this way!"

The man was reflective. "Is this . . . frog kissing?" he asked.

"Wonderful!" shouted John. "You've got it! That's it!"

Again the man was quiet and thoughtful. Frog kissing was something more than a cute little phrase. The idea had many implications. "This extends to other areas of life, doesn't it?" asked the man.

"It surely does." John smiled. "Frog kissing has unlimited applications! Some people feel they are married to a frog! Some think they work for a frog. Some people see everybody else in the world as a frog."

Both men laughed.

"But those are just the windows of approval, judgment, and expectation that guarantee we will never know the power of love. I changed my entire experience of life when I realized that other people do not have to change for me to love them. Instead, I have to change for me to love them! Isn't that a revolutionary thought?"

❧❧❧

Other people do not have to change

for me to love them.

I have to change

for me to love them.

❧❧❧

John jumped to his feet and waved his arms. "Our first job is to go from faultfinder to lovefinder—of ourselves and of others. We can make that choice. It depends on us! It's within our control. Isn't that wonderful? Instead of judging we can live, laugh, and love. Isn't that a happy and hopeful thought?"

The man smiled. You felt a sense of joy seeing John wave his arms exuberantly and hearing him talk about love in his booming voice. And the man had to admit, there was hope in this frog-kissing message. How refreshing. We didn't have to judge everyone! Or ourselves. Going from fault-finder to lovefinder—this was a very good thing!

"There's a happiness in this outlook, isn't there?" asked the man. "Frog kissing leads to joy, doesn't it?"

"You're terrific!" said John. "I can see you're going to conquer your cancer because you're so open to these principles. You've already grasped the next step in *live*—joy! With love there comes happiness. And with happiness, joy is possible.

"You know, inside each of us is a child—the good, non-manipulative, fun-loving, filled-with-joy little person who needs to be nourished. The Cancer Conqueror believes that most cancer patients have failed for years to appropriately nurture this inner child. And by not honoring the child's real needs, they may be contributing to their illness or inhibiting their recovery.

"I used to deny the needs of my child," said John. "I always felt that those needs were far behind me. After all, I had matured. I had grown. I didn't need to laugh and play. Or so I thought. Wow, was I wrong! My needs to honor my inner child are very strong. I'll bet you have those same needs."

The man said, "I'm not sure. Tell me more."

"There are two parts to finding joy. The first is an issue of attitude. To me, joy is giving life a big hug, embracing all the beauty and wonder and goodness there is in this world. Joy is not how much you possess but how much you enjoy.

❧❧

Joy is not

how much you possess

but how much you enjoy.

❧❧

"I once saw a bumper sticker that said, 'The one with the most toys wins!' My suggestion is 'The one with the most joys wins.' It's that attitude that looks for joy in the small, precious packages and makes the most of them, knowing that the big packages of joy are really few and far between."

"That sounds intriguing!" said the man. "I wish I were able to capture more of those moments."

"You can," said John. "You see, the second part of finding joy, of letting the inner child come out, is action. Simply put, we need to allow time for play."

"Play?" questioned the man.

"Yes, play." John smiled. "That kid inside needs time to play every day."

"But play sounds so . . . so . . . I guess it seems child-ish," said the man.

"That's the idea!" retorted John. "That's just what we're looking for—ways to nurture that inner child. This can become an important step in your recovery journey. The idea is to have fun, to create an enjoyable experience. The person who can find joy and laughter will be much better off than the stoic person who seldom cracks a smile and won't acknowledge his or her feelings. That's what you saw me doing when you walked in today. That jug-gling is one of my forms of play. And far from taking away from my capacity for work, it actually helps increase my energy for living, for healing.

"When I first heard the Cancer Conqueror talk about laughter and play, I assumed it wasn't for me. I had a cer-tain rigidity about releasing the inner child. Then the Cancer Conqueror talked about messages we may have learned as children. Her ideas really hit home.

"Early in life I was conditioned to 'try hard,' 'be seri-ous,' 'be strong,' 'be successful,' 'be a good provider.' And I've heard women describe their messages to 'be perfect,' 'please others,' 'nurture everyone,' 'look nice.' When I realized how I'd been conditioned, I came to understand that I allowed no room for play. Do you know what I did? I actually had to start out by giving myself an assignment. I had to schedule time to play. Isn't that crazy?"

The man shook his head. "No, not at all. I find it refresh-ing. This cancer journey has once again confronted me with me. That's exactly the way I am. I learned the same things. I have the same attitudes toward play that you did."

"Well, you can change just as I did," said John. "First, I gave myself permission to play. I made play a more important part of my life. I used to say, 'I'll play after work.' Well, the work is never done. Now I treat work and play with the same attitude—both are important. Both deserve my best. I decided that play is okay.

"The next thing I did may seem even more childish, but it was most helpful. I gave my inner child a name! As a youngster, nobody called me John. I was known by my nickname, Buddy. I always liked that. So I started calling my inner child Buddy. It's great! I still do it! At first I asked my inner child what he needed to get well. And today I ask Buddy what he needs to stay well.

"A helpful perspective for me was when the Cancer Conqueror suggested that we think of the part of us that got cancer as this inner child. Then an important part of our task becomes taking care of that child, nurturing the child back to health, helping the child conquer cancer. So when I ask Buddy what he needs to stay well, I'm trying to get in touch with myself attitudinally, emotionally, and behaviorally on a very foundational level. Buddy invariably wants me to honor his needs to experience laughter, play, and joy. I listen. I now honor those needs." John smiled again.

"That's special how you talk with your inner child. I'm going to do that today!" said the man. "I've often sensed some of these things, but I never really talked to my child. This sounds exciting."

"When you talk to your inner child," said John, "you might want to do what the Cancer Conqueror suggests. She had me write down fifty different things I could do, actual activities I felt would bring me fun and produce joy in my life. Just try that exercise. It was difficult for me to find fifty items at first. I suppose my child was so undernourished that he had forgotten how to play. But now my list has more than a hundred and fifty activities—and it's still increasing."

"That's wonderful," said the man. "But I think I'm going to have trouble coming up with even ten ways to play."

"You'll learn," said John. "I found that it was important for me just to block out the time to play. In the beginning there were some days that I didn't do a thing. But just scheduling the time was most helpful. And soon I began to fill that time with enjoyable activities.

"Once I heard the Cancer Conqueror talk about play in conjunction with treatments. A woman dreaded going in for radiation treatments. So the Cancer Conqueror had her sandwich the treatments between play. Before she went in, she scheduled thirty minutes of piano playing for herself. And afterward, she went window-shopping, just to treat herself to the sights and senses. Interesting. Her dread of the treatments decreased, and the side effects she was experiencing completely disappeared. She was now taking care of her inner child.

"So, nurture your inner child," continued John. "Play is much more than an activity; it is an attitude that generates energy for healing. And notice you're never too tired to play. If we think we are tired, perhaps it's the strongest signal that we need play now. Honor your inner child's fundamental needs."

"Thanks for giving me permission to play," said the man. He chuckled. "You know, I already feel better. Just the idea of frog kissing, maybe that's even better! I'm going to become a positive, passionate, playful frog kisser! How about that?"

Both men laughed out loud! Perhaps it was the mental picture that a playful frog kisser conjured up. At any rate, there was significant release in their laughter—a safety valve opened.

Then John spoke again. "It's wonderful to see you laugh and smile and express that joy in your eyes. Yet as healthy and healing as being a playful frog kisser might be, there's something ever better."

"What is that?" asked the man.

"Well, all the love in our hearts, all the joy in the world, resolving all our problems, even changing all our beliefs, is empty without one essential ingredient. I once heard a person describe it this way. All our efforts are like a long string of zeros. They mean nothing without a digit in front of them. That digit is peace of mind."

The man was quiet.

"You see, peace is the ultimate destination of the conquering cancer journey. The goal is to create peace of mind, not just to cure cancer.

❧❧

The goal is to create

peace of mind,

not just to cure cancer.

❧❧

"Personal peace creates an environment conducive to healing the body, mind, and spirit. Peace is perhaps the finest way to allow the body's powerful healing mechanisms to function."

"Okay," said the man, "I like what you're saying, but really what is personal peace? And how do I go about achieving it?"

"Good questions," said John. "I like the definition the Cancer Conqueror teaches: 'Personal peace is transcending oneself in order to nurture inner harmony.' Let's give this definition a closer look.

"First, personal peace is transcending. The idea is that personal peace requires intent and choice and action. It is not some chance occurrence. And personal peace transcends self—meaning that the decision is consciously made to set aside self-limitations of fear, anger, and guilt and to rest upon the unshakable foundation of spiritual tranquillity that lies within each of us. Resting on that foundation, there is our goal."

"I don't hear you talking about outer quietness," said the man.

"Many people would include that," said John, "and others would not. For me, personal peace includes times of outer quietness as well as times of activity. The Cancer Conqueror really takes peace out of the activity realm when she says, 'You will know personal peace when what you think, what you say, and what you do are essentially consistent.' I believe this is what we're really after, an inner consistency. Quietness may play a part. But so does activity.

"You see, it isn't so much the physical aspects as it is the inner aspects, the emotional and spiritual components, that make for personal peace. This is especially important for the cancer patient. When we realize that peace of mind is independent from our physical condition, true healing has begun."

❧❧

Peace of mind is independent from our physical condition.

❧❧

There was a pause. "Ah-ha," said the man. "A lightbulb has just gone on in my mind. Personal peace brings it all together, doesn't it?"

John nodded his agreement.

"How do I achieve this peace? How do I work to make this a way of life?"

John stood, stretched, and walked across the office. "You know," he began, "of all the changes the Cancer Conqueror encouraged me to make, the daily pursuit of personal peace has had the single most dramatic effect on my outer and inner life. If there was one change I could point to that most altered my daily schedule, one with the greatest potential for healing, it would be this pursuit—seeking the profound personal peace that is available to all of us. I do practice quiet time, a daily dose of tranquillity, that gets me in touch with the deeper levels of personal peace that are always waiting there for me to access."

The man looked a bit puzzled. "This seems a little far out. What do you mean?"

John smiled that reassuring grin as he sat down. "Just listen with an open mind. There is so much healing potential here. Twice each day, I set aside fifteen minutes to calm my mind, examine my spirit, and affirm my total well-being in all areas of my life. Here at work, at home, when I travel, wherever I am, I find or make a quiet spot where I won't be disturbed. Twice each day—more if I am dealing with lot of stress—I still my spirit, affirm my well-being, and find personal peace.

"I sit in a comfortable position, close my eyes, and first turn my attention to the physical tension in my body. I take special care to consciously relax my muscles from head to feet, particularly those in the shoulders, neck, and forehead. One of my biggest revelations was my jaw—I was always clenching it and gritting my teeth, pushing my tongue up against the roof of my mouth. No wonder I was always getting headaches. From the shoulders up, I was one knot of tense muscles. I now take time to consciously relax this area."

The man followed John's suggestion. He took a deep breath, tensed his neck and shoulder muscles, and, as he exhaled, consciously released all the muscle tension through his entire body. He relaxed, his muscles limp. It felt safe, and good.

"Next, I conceive of my mind as the surface of a body of water. I have the mental picture of a lake. And when I think of the stress and tension that have been part of my day, I see the surface of the lake churning with whitecaps. But then I imagine changing the scene, having the power to make those waves dissipate. I make the lake's undulating surface calm—

placid and smooth, just like a mirror. At the same time I repeat the word *peace* silently in time with my breathing.

"Amazingly, not only does my mind follow with thoughts that are calming and soothing but my whole spirit feels a weight lifted. When a stressful thought or worry comes to mind, I gently dismiss it and make my thoughts go right back to the calm, smooth surface of that lake and to my focus word, *peace*."

The man smiled. "I like what you're suggesting. It's all so peaceful."

"Wonderful," said John. "That tells me you can easily and effectively do this exercise. Remember, the goal is first to relax the muscles. This, in itself, is a healing experience and will help in your total wellness. Then calm the mind. Dismiss the random thoughts that come and return to the placid, peaceful serenity you have found.

"I also use this as an opportunity to examine my spirit and to listen for the deeper messages of harmony found in quieting the mind. Many thoughts that cross my mind in my internal dialogue have to do with judging and with feeling that I have to be right. When I observe my spirit, I ask if those thoughts are bringing me love, joy, and peace. Invariably it is a revealing and growing experience. I listen to my inner self. Some call this intuition. Others call it conscience, inner wisdom, or the subconscious. I just think of it as my inner self.

"I ask the questions like 'Am I creating love, joy, and peace?' Then I wait for my inner response. 'Is my marriage reflecting love, joy, and peace?' 'What about my vocation? My physical well-being? My relationships? Our finances? My self-development?' The idea is to examine the important areas of life, listening for the guidance of my inner wisdom. When I get a positive response, I'm thankful for it and I express gratitude. When I hear a negative response, I ask, 'What is the message? How do I need to change?' With practice, I was able to get on speaking terms with my inner self. I now feel this inner guidance is a highly important part of my life."

"How do you know you're not just selfishly creating answers you want to hear?" asked the man.

"Excellent question. You see, I truly believe that love, joy, and peace are supremely important in life. If I receive signals that are based in fear, anger, and guilt, I know I need to change; I need to let go again. If I receive answers based in love, joy, and peace, I trust them because they are consistent with my aim."

"But when you say, 'Let go,' what do you mean?" wondered the man.

"You've asked a profound question that has been asked through the ages. To me," continued John, "letting go means adopting an attitude of relaxed trust. Relaxed trust is that sense of inner harmony—that serenity and peacefulness—that comes from knowing all is well, even if you have cancer. You can let go. You don't have to judge. You don't have to approve. You don't have to control. You don't have to be right every moment. You can give yourself a vacation from trying to be Manager of the Universe!"

Both men laughed. How often they both had tried to assume that role. New thinking was required.

"Daily examining, observing, listening—those are guideposts on the path of wellness," John went on. "And this leads to the final part of my daily quiet time—affirming myself. Many people use affirmations to replace old, ingrained thinking patterns. Positive phrases, repeated often and with emotion, can lead to new understanding. They help counter conditioned thinking. Affirmations help change our beliefs about cancer. The end of your quiet time is an appropriate time for these affirmations.

"But there is another side to affirmations. This has to do with affirming—some would say directing, others might say rehearsing—your body's own natural healing capacities. The idea of mental reviews of desired activities is well-accepted. One example is Olympic athletes who regularly employ creative imagination to gain a competitive edge. For example, the more an athlete imagines a successful jump over the crossbar, the more deeply etched the mental and emotional circuits become. In short, we tend to become what we think about."

"Exactly what are you suggesting?" questioned the man.

John looked him squarely in the eyes. "I am suggesting that you have significant control over your immune system, your natural defense against cancer."

"Is this more of the psychoneuroimmunology I've previously studied?" asked the man.

"It is," said John. "And the primary technique for consciously stimulating our immune system is using creative imagination during our daily quiet time. One researcher called it healing with brain chemistry. Our immune defenses tend to weaken under stress. Quiet time with relaxation exercises and creative imagination may be one of the best ways to better manage the biochemical results of stress. We thus keep our resistance high."

"Do I hear you saying that in addition to my emotions

influencing my immune system, I can also consciously enhance the functioning of my immune system?"

John spoke firmly and with deep conviction. "I am saying that creatively and consciously imagining our immune system functioning effectively may indeed enhance it. I am also recognizing that the immune system may be positively triggered as the roadblocks of fear, anger, and guilt are replaced with love, joy, and peace. And I am suggesting that as we imagine malignant cells being eliminated, and as we imagine ourselves as healthy, whole, and feeling well, our entire being—body, mind, and spirit—will move in the direction of health. That is something we cherish and for which we can strive!"

"I've heard of this before," said the man. "But I'm afraid I am a skeptic. A positive attitude is one thing. But the mind actually have physiological effects—I don't think so."

"I'm sorry you feel that way," said John. "Would you try an experiment with me here and now? Would you be willing to see if we could trigger a system in our body with only our thoughts?"

"Sure, I'm willing to try. What do we do?"

John made himself comfortable, reclining slightly in his chair and stretching his legs out. He invited the man to do the same. "Okay, now just close your eyes. Keep them closed. Imagine yourself in your kitchen. Go to the refrigerator, where you find a big, yellow lemon. As you hold the bright, firm lemon, run your fingers over the texture of its skin. Feel the shape. See the color. Lift it to your nose and smell its sharp, pungent odor.

"Now walk over to the counter, where you find a paring knife. Cut the lemon in half. Notice the spray as you cut this juicy lemon. And cut one of the halves in half.

Smell the aroma as the juice runs over your fingers. Now take one of the wedges of the lemon and bring it right to your nose. Deeply inhale the fragrance. Now, put the lemon wedge right between your teeth. Bite down hard. Taste the strangely tart juices as they roll over your tongue and throughout your mouth."

"Okay, okay!" The man laughed. "You've made your point. I can't believe the amount of saliva that produces!"

"The fact is," said John, "the body cannot tell the difference between what is actually taking place and what you are imagining is taking place. This principle is at the very heart of what I was saying about the vital importance of imagining our immune systems functioning effectively. Does this example do anything to shift your thinking about this being some sort of deception?"

"Well, I have visualized many times before. I used it in my work. I know it works there. Perhaps it will work here. Tell me, how did you go about enhancing your immune system?" said the man.

"My method was to see my cancer as something weak, and my immune system as something strong that would easily have the ability to handle the cancer. And during my treatment period, I imagined the treatment as effective, a strong friend who was there to help rid my body of cancer."

"Yes, but how did you know what a cancer cell looks like? And the same for your immune system and the treatment?"

John gave a chuckle. "You know what I did? I gave them all symbols. I didn't know the anatomy of cancer cells or the biochemical properties of treatments. I was told that sort of technical knowledge was not important.

It wasn't even critical that I knew where the cancer was located. What was important is that I imagined my immune system and treatment as being effective. So I imagined my cancer as ice cubes. And I saw my immune system as hot water. I viewed radiation therapy as an intense ray of white-hot light. The hot water and the ray of light melted the ice, and the cancer was flushed from my body naturally. This was a most effective image for me.

"You'll discover your own images. Just choose a weak image for the cancer and strong images for both your immune system and your treatment. And 'see' the damaged cancer cells flushed from your body, normally and naturally. Then, end your quiet time by affirming yourself as healthy and free from cancer. This isn't self-deception. It's self-direction. And it moves us in the direction of wellness. Now, what do you think about using your creative imagination?" asked John.

"Well, I'm going to try it. I can't help but believe in its potential. I've seen the principle work in other areas of my life. So I'm going to put it to use here."

"There's one more important thing that needs to be said," John added. "Engaging in creative imagination and affirming our own healing capabilities are different from quieting our minds and examining our spirits. Creative imagination is goal-directed. We actively guide our imaginations. Quieting our minds and examining our spirits are observation-directed. They help us become more aware of thoughts and choices. They aid us in deciding to let go of those things that hold us back."

"Which is more important?" asked the man.

"Both have a role. Realize that we aren't simply imagining our immune system attacking cancer cells. Instead, we are seeking to move our entire being—body, mind, and spirit—in the direction of wellness.

❧❧❧

We are moving

our entire being—

body, mind, and spirit—

in the direction of wellness.

❧❧❧

"I am suggesting that as important as your creative imagination can be, consider it as an adjunct to the pursuit of daily quiet times. I suggest that you keep as your most important goal the quieting of the mind and examining of the spirit. The new awareness gained here is what you seek. It generates peace of mind!"

The man finished his notes. "We've covered a lot of material."

John smiled that special smile once again. "We have! But that's it, my friend. That's *live*. Live, laugh, and love! To be a peaceful, playful frog kisser! That's your aim, and it's also the essence of health!"

The men stood. John put his hands on the man's shoulders and looked straight into his eyes. "Now go and live your life one moment at a time. You can never tell when the greatest moment of your life is going to happen. So go and live each moment as if it were the greatest—the greatest to live, laugh, and love."

The men embraced. "Thank you," said the man. He left feeling at peace with himself and the world.

As soon as the man was home, he sat down at his desk and summarized his notes.

Live *Summary*

1. Unconditional love conquers cancer.
2. Healing has at its roots the ability to give and receive unconditional love.
3. My task is to accept others, not approve of others.
4. Other people do not have to change for me to love them. I have to change for me to love them.
5. Joy is not how much I possess but how much I enjoy.
6. Play is okay. Make a list of fifty activities that are fun, that bring me joy.
7. Acknowledge my inner child. Ask, "What do you need to get well?"
8. The goal is to create peace of mind not just to cure cancer. Peace of mind creates an environment conducive to healing.
9. Peace of mind is independent from my physical condition.
10. Schedule quiet time—at least fifteen minutes twice a day:

    ❦ Consciously relax my muscles from head to feet.
    ❦ Focus thoughts on a peaceful scene, dismissing other thoughts as they come. Return to that peaceful place.

❧ Listen to my inner self, being thankful for love, joy, and peace and being open to messages to change.
❧ Affirm myself and my immune system working to overcome the cancer.

❧ Author's Encouragement ❧

No matter how you are feeling, I ask you to consider the following exercises now.

❧ LIVE: ❧
NURTURING A SENSE OF JOY

Cancer takes a cumulative toll on our lives. It is an unparalleled dilemma that threatens our personal security and erodes our sense of spontaneity. We feel angry at our misfortune and usually have ample evidence to conclude that life is unfair.

The crisis of cancer explodes many of the illusions that once anchored our lives. After we have been told we have cancer, it makes little difference if our home is perfectly neat and clean. Being critically ill overrides all concern with meeting sales quotas or updating quarterly financial projections.

Cancer makes it easy for us to slip into despair. The threat is all too real; the changes rock our personal foundations. Life feels so out of control. Helplessness is often the simplest way to cope. It is not the best way.

An alternate response can lead us to a new era in our lives. This new era is characterized by joyfulness. However, it requires our choice coupled with our fortitude; it is an intentional choice. For in the midst of this crisis, we can learn what is important, and we can act on what will be the redemptive legacy of this unwanted experience. In short, we can learn to live.

Joy, the sense of well-being evoked by an awareness that life is truly a special gift, is central to our understanding. Joy is delight in life no matter what the circumstances. Joy is personal peace coupled with a liberal sprinkling of bliss. Joy is the experience of happiness even in the face of life-threatening illness. Joy is what it means to live.

"Cancering" can be seen as a testing of our spirits. The following exercises focus on increasing our awareness of joy, the essential fortification we need in response to cancer. These queries will help you understand what you define as truly joyful and thus important.

Cultivate Joyfulness

Consider each statement. Indicate your level of agreement by circling the relative value from 10 to 1. Reflect on your level of intensity—always, often, sometimes, seldom, or never—surrounding each choice.

❈ I appreciate optimism and its contribution to my well-being.

Always		Often		Sometimes		Seldom		Never	
10	9	8	7	6	5	4	3	2	1

Thought Starters: List three actions that nearly always help you feel optimistic and hopeful. List three thought patterns that nearly always elicit pessimism and despair.

_____

_____

_____

_____

_____

_____

_____

_____

_____

_____

_____

_____

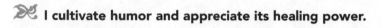 **I cultivate humor and appreciate its healing power.**

Always		*Often*		*Sometimes*		*Seldom*		*Never*
10	9	8	7	6	5	4	3	2	1

Thought Starters: What triggers my deep and genuine laughter? How might I access those moments more frequently?

_____

_____

_____

_____

_____

_____

_____

_____

_____

≫ I regularly enjoy a variety of playful activities that are both relaxing and rejuvenating.

Always		Often		Sometimes		Seldom		Never	
10	9	8	7	6	5	4	3	2	1

Thought Starters:

≫ List ten playful activities that cost nothing.

_____

_____

_____

_____

_____

_____

_____

_____

_____

_____

≫ List ten playful activities that cost under five dollars each.

_____

_____

_____

_____

_____

_____

_____

_____

_____

_____

❧ **List ten playful activities that involve a partner.**

_____

_____

_____

_____

_____

_____

_____

_____

_____

❧ **List ten playful activities that involve art or culture.**

_____

_____

_____

_____

_____

_____

_____

_____

_____

_____

❧ **List ten playful activities that involve volunteer service to others.**

_____

_____

_____

_____

_____

_____

_____

_____

_____

_____

_____

_____

_____

_____

I give and get as much touching and hugging as I need.

Always		Often		Sometimes		Seldom		Never
10	9	8	7	6	5	4	3	2	1

Thought Starters: What "rules of displaying affection" did my family of origin live by? Do I practice the same as an adult? Should I make any changes in my "rules"? Do I feel the freedom to be openly expressive?

❧ **I am playful in my close relationships, laughing at myself and others about our shared foibles.**

Always	Often		Sometimes		Seldom		Never	
10	9	8	7	6	5	4	3	2	1

Thought Starters: List three ways playful love was expressed in your family of origin. Do you practice the same as an adult? Should you make any changes in your expression?

_____

_____

_____

_____

_____

_____

_____

_____

_____

_____

_____

_____

_____

_____

❧ **I enjoy and affirm my own strengths, accomplishments, and successes as well as those of others.**

Always		Often		Sometimes		Seldom		Never	
10	9	8	7	6	5	4	3	2	1

Thought Starters: List three examples of your affirmative self-talk. List three examples of your critical self-talk. How can you shift away from the negative and increase the positive affirmations in your life?

_____

_____

_____

_____

_____

_____

_____

_____

_____

_____

_____

_____

_____

_____

❧ I allow myself to give love openly.

Always		Often		Sometimes		Seldom		Never	
10	9	8	7	6	5	4	3	2	1

Thought Starters: List five ways you give love effectively and to whom. Note whether any expectations of return are attached to your love giving. How do you benefit from your expressions of love?

✖ I allow myself to openly receive love.

Always	Often	Sometimes	Seldom	Never
10 9	8 7	6 5	4 3	2 1

Thought Starters: What mental picture do you hold of being loved? Where do you turn to fulfill that need? When human love temporarily fails you, how do you respond?

❧ I am able to sustain hope and joy even when cancer seems to dictate otherwise.

Always		Often		Sometimes		Seldom		Never	
10	9	8	7	6	5	4	3	2	1

Thought Starters: What are your hopes? Where can you turn to find a constant personal wellspring of hope? How much time do you spend in seeking this source?

_____

_____

_____

_____

_____

_____

_____

_____

_____

_____

_____

_____

_____

_____

_____

_____

❧ **I am able to allow vital well-being to radiate from me, even when cancer would block my light.**

Always   *Often*   *Sometimes*   *Seldom*   *Never*

10   9   8   7   6   5   4   3   2   1

Thought Starters: What does it mean for you to radiate wellness? If your wellness was a lightbulb, how brightly would that light be shining now?

_____

_____

_____

_____

_____

_____

_____

_____

_____

_____

_____

_____

_____

_____

_____

For the Advanced Wellness Student

Cancer recovery takes appropriate downtime, moments when we do nothing more constructive than honor our own needs. This does not mean a permanent retreat into isolation and loneliness. Instead, downtime prepares us to live. If we deprive ourselves of this necessity, we soon become like caged animals; at first we snarl at our family and friends, even God. But soon we become resigned to "the inevitable" and give in to the despair.

Advanced wellness students recognize and stop such behavior. I give you permission to claim all the downtime you need. Create the unique feelings of joy and satisfaction that are distinctive to your own recovery. Above all, give yourself the necessary permission to live, laugh, and love—it's as simple as changing a thought.

Many cancer patients have made a virtue out of deprivation. We sacrifice for others. We constantly put our own needs second or third. Sometimes, we've used a long-suffering stance in life to feed a false sense of our spirituality. We've served others to the point of disservice to ourselves. In doing so, we've called ourselves good and at moments may even have claimed some moral superiority for these acts. Cancer is calling you to step out of that behavior. We stay there because we feel like listless circus animals who are regularly prodded to perform. And if we perform, we receive some applause and earn our daily bread.

Come out. Live. Laugh. Love. Do not be afraid to appear selfish. Heal yourself by saying yes to your true self. Anything less is being self-destructive. Are you self-destructive? This is a very delicate question to answer with accuracy because it requires that we know something of who we really are. And that is a person whom many cancer patients have long ago forced into the proverbial circus cage.

Who are you, really? One quick way to get a sense is to ask yourself this question:

❧ **What would I try if it wasn't viewed as crazy by others? List the things you would like to do, achieve, or be if you could.**

_____

_____

_____

_____

_____

_____

_____

_____

_____

_____

_____

If your list looks pretty exciting, even a bit crazy, then you are on the right track. These are actually voices about living from one's true self. They are less about being selfish and more about honoring the real you. I asked one of our Cancer Recovery classes to share their lists. Items included:

- ❧ Learn to waltz
- ❧ Sail the entire Mediterranean
- ❧ Participate in an archaeological dig
- ❧ Spend a week at a health spa
- ❧ Take voice and acting lessons
- ❧ Buy a Corvette convertible
- ❧ Locate my first true love
- ❧ Finish my college degree
- ❧ Move to Colorado
- ❧ Become a missionary in Sudan

Check your own list. Don't neglect this important work. Seek to understand what lies hidden within and then embrace the possibilities for making that real. Then you will achieve new levels of well-being. This is not an easy task. To help focus your imagination, complete the following prompts with the first thoughts that come to your mind.

❧ The most significant lack in my life is

_____

_____

_____

_____

_____

_____

❧ **My most significant time commitment is**

_____

_____

_____

_____

_____

_____

❧ **One reason I become fearful is**

_____

_____

_____

_____

_____

_____

❧ **One reason I get angry is**

_____

_____

_____

_____

_____

_____

❧ **One reason I feel guilty is**

_____

_____

_____

_____

_____

_____

❧ **One reason I become sad is**

_____

_____

_____

_____

_____

❧ **As I play more, my work**

_____

_____

_____

_____

_____

_____

❧ **I sometimes sabotage myself by**

_____

_____

_____

_____

_____

❧ **If my dreams really came true, my family would**

_____

_____

_____

_____

_____

_____

❧ **The greatest joy in my life is**

_____

_____

_____

_____

_____

_____

One reason this is such a difficult exercise to complete with integrity is the cultural expectations we have accepted without question. A grandmother once shared that the greatest joy in her life was her grandchildren. In the next breath she told how much she resented postponing her own activities to once again baby-sit while her daughter and son-in-law went out. Saying no to her daughter would be saying yes to herself. Unfortunately, it was a responsibility the grandmother couldn't manage. One of the central questions of healing becomes Am I regularly honoring my own true needs? It definitely is not Am I meeting the expectations of others?

Resolve today to *live!* One of the best ways to become more aware of our true needs is to silence our "internal critics" through a simple technique called speed writing. Here, we respond quickly to a series of prompts. And since wishes are just wishes and are allowed to be frivolous, we can feel free to express them.

❧ As quickly as you can, finish the following phrases:

I wish _____

_____

I wish _____

_____

I wish _____

_____

I wish _____

_____

I wish _____

_____

I wish _____

_____

I wish _____

_____

I wish _____

_____

I wish _____

_____

I wish _____

_____

I wish _____

_____

I wish _____

_____

I wish _____

_____

I wish _____

_____

I wish _____

_____

I wish _____

_____

I wish _____

_____

I wish _____

_____

I wish _____

_____

I especially wish _____

_____

_____

Wishes should frequently be taken seriously. Circle those that fall into the "take them seriously" category for you.

FROG KISSING. What was your reaction to the frog-kissing story? Do you believe giving and receiving unconditional love can conquer cancer? On what level?

_____

_____

_____

_____

_____

_____

_____

_____

_____

_____

_____

_____

_____

One of the most important things you can do for your recovery and well-being is to nurture healthy love in your closest relationships. When all else is done, our intimate relationships help us get well, stay well, and transcend the frightening experience of cancer. Your recovery is inherently and inescapably bound to your relationships. As much as I have encouraged you to have a sense of autonomy and meet your own needs, this is done to facilitate your deep need to relate authentically with others. This need to give and receive love is the most basic of our heart hungers. Honor it. Make a list of those dear ones—your inner circle of mutual caring and love.

Who are the people to whom you would most like to say, "I love you"?

_____

_____

_____

_____

_____

_____

_____

_____

_____

_____

_____

❦ **To whom do you wish to say, "Thank you?"**

_____

_____

_____

_____

_____

_____

_____

_____

_____

_____

Now, before you do anything else, express your feelings to each of these people. Do so face-to-face, by phone, through a handwritten note, or via E-mail. Tell them what you want them to know about your feelings toward them. Bask in the well-being.

🙣 6 🙡

Cancer
Conquerors
Transcend

The man felt exceptional. John's *live* message gave him hope! He called the Cancer Conqueror the very next morning. "I've completed the assignments," he said. They scheduled a meeting that afternoon, right after the man's appointment with his doctor.

When the man arrived at the Cancer Conqueror's home, his mood had changed. The Cancer Conqueror picked up on the change immediately. "Compared to our phone call this morning, you seem troubled. Do you need to talk?"

"Yes, I do, and I'll tell you exactly what it is," said the man. "I've just come from my oncologist's office. And while I'm doing great, just seeing all those patients in that waiting room wasn't a good experience. It's depressing! I talked with a woman who had just experienced a recurrence. It's a frightening prospect to work at getting well only to have the cancer return."

"Wait! Slow down!" said the Cancer Conqueror. "You're awfulizing, you're letting your thoughts assume the worst possible outcomes. Admittedly, an oncology office is not the best place to seek a lift. You see people there who are hurting, who are feeling hopeless and overwhelmed. When I have to schedule an appointment with my oncologist, I first become aware that I'll need to toughen myself mentally. And one of the issues is the people in the waiting room. I'm probably going to see some emaciated folks. Just looking at them can cause me to question myself and my own beliefs.

"But realizing this is helpful. If I am feeling strong emotionally, I often make an effort to sit beside someone who looks especially needy. My goal is then to give whatever word of encouragement I can honestly muster. I try to take a negative and turn it into something positive. And when I do, invariably I feel better. I've come to understand the truth that you cannot help another person without helping yourself."

"Okay," said the man. "I understand what you're suggesting. But the fact is, I talked to a woman who was cancer-free for seven years. Now it's back! The idea of a recurrence always haunting me is frightening."

The Cancer Conqueror was firm. "The fact is, the possibility of recurrence will always be with you. The course of the disease is uncertain. Even so, there is a reason for hope. There is a pervasive belief that is behind almost all worries of recurrence. The belief goes something like, 'Yes, I may battle the cancer with some success, but in the end the biological process will win and it will eventually get me.' Have you ever heard that?"

"Sure, just today I heard that from the woman who had the recurrence."

"That belief is a major untruth. It is reasonably common for people to go into remission, have a recurrence, and eventually enjoy recovery. Once again, the importance of our beliefs comes into play. We must first understand that recurrence does not mean imminent death.

❧❧

Recurrence does not mean imminent death.

❧❧

"Yet, we need to treat recurrence as a crisis. For some people, this is obvious. Their pain is significant, or perhaps they can actually feel or see tumor growth. And it is common for fear to be more intense with recurrence. People may also feel out of control and lose faith in their medical team, their treatment, as well as the entire program they have been implementing. Feelings like 'I've failed' and 'I give up' are common. That's probably what you saw this morning with that woman."

"That was precisely it," said the man. "And it scares me."

"I've gone through recurrence," said the Cancer Conqueror. "It was frightening. But I did some things that made it a turning point. Consider this same strategy for yourself.

First, I treated myself very gently. I had been back at work, but now I took more time off. I scheduled a vacation at one of our favorite places. And I spent time alone, time to reflect.

"I talked with others, people who successfully overcame the illness. It was helpful to understand that many of them also went through recurrence. Almost all used recurrence as a time to reevaluate. So I followed their advice. I went back to the medical team and had the doctors review the recent evaluations in detail and answer my questions. This helped.

"Then I reviewed my beliefs about illness and recovery, examined the major emotional conflicts still present in my life, and looked more closely at what I could do to bring more joy and well-being into my life. Finally, I asked an important question of myself. Did I want to work toward health once again, or did I want to accept death and spend my energy preparing for it? You can see which I chose—I was willing once again to work toward recovery."

"But what if you had died? There weren't any guarantees that you would recover," said the man.

"Not one," said the Cancer Conqueror. "But guarantees aren't the issue. I said that I would work toward recovery, that I would strive for health. I could only work toward them. I had to realize that even though I don't control my destiny, I do influence it. And I chose to influence it toward health."

❧❧

Even though I don't control

my destiny, I do influence it.

❧❧

The man finished his notes and looked up. "I need something with a lot more certainty. I am expecting this program to bring me health."

"It can," said the Cancer Conqueror. "But are you also saying that you'll reject it if it doesn't meet all your expectations? If so, I can't help you. I can't give you any guarantee. I can only share that for me it was—and still is—a hill-and-valley experience. I refused to view the valley of recurrence as a failure. Instead, I chose to see recurrence as a message. I needed once again to understand the message and decide what my response would be.

"For me the message of recurrence was clearly that I was not taking care of myself as I needed to. Up to that time, I was not really following the diet I knew was best for me. I was exercising only occasionally. I wasn't taking time to play. I only sporadically worked with my creative imagination. And I only partially resolved some of the emotional turmoil that still raged in my life. When I honestly looked at myself, I realized that I had, in many ways, returned to the lifestyle that contributed to my initial illness. I came to understand that recurrence was my body's way of telling me to choose to change again."

The man was uneasy. "Maybe the real issue of recurrence with me is the possibility that death is near. That scares me so much. I don't want to die. It's all so frightening."

"Okay," said the Cancer Conqueror. "Let's talk about death. When you think about death, what is it that you most fear?"

"Oh, no," said the man pensively. "The whole thing is so frightening. First, I don't even like to think about it. Maybe it's the fear of lying there helpless, not being able to take care of myself. I don't want to be an invalid. And the people we leave behind. That's sad. And it's also this emptiness about no longer existing. I get depressed just thinking that it's all going to come to an end."

"Then let's face this fear," said the Cancer Conqueror. "Instead of saying we don't want to deal with an issue, let's take the fear of death and start to transcend it right now. Look at what you said. You fear three things about death. One is the issue of being an invalid. That has to do with the process of dying, the quality of death. And you also said you felt sad about leaving. That has to do with severing our earthly ties. Finally you said you felt empty about no longer existing. This is the issue of what may or may not come after death."

"Yes." The man sighed. "That's it."

"There is so much we don't know about death," said the Cancer Conqueror. "But surprisingly, there is much we do know; a great deal has been written about it. I encourage you to seek out the resources you need. But today, let's not make it our aim to fully explore death. Instead, let's just attempt to help you through the basic issue of facing your own fear of death.

"I remember discussing the issue of death with a pastor. In a blinding flash of the obvious he said, 'First, I assume you believe you will die. I mean, the statistics are overwhelming! A thousand out of a thousand people die! There don't seem to be many exceptions!' The implications of his humor hit me immediately. Of course I would die. The question wasn't if; the question was when and how.

"Most people are anxious about death's when and how. There is sadness and possibly anger over the prospect of a shortened life—the when. Perhaps there are dreams still to pursue and people still to love. So a shortened life span seems unfair.

"Yet in a very real sense, people live on in the memories of others. If we want to guarantee a loving memory, if we want to guarantee that we accomplished something significant with our lives, then we need to love, and love now! That's the secret to overcoming the fear of death's when— it's to love now, today, this hour, while we have the opportunity. The key point of understanding is to realize that our life's value is measured not by its duration but by its donations—of love."

❧❧

A life's value

is measured not by its duration

but by its donations—

of love.

❧❧

The man nodded. "Yes. That's very helpful," he said. "And profound."

"And then there is the dread of a low quality of death. A long, debilitating illness that could drain the family and the patient emotionally and financially is the real fear. This is the unpleasant how part, a fear that there is little control over death.

"Unlike many causes of death, cancer usually allows ample time to prepare. This preparation and taking control can be very comforting. Some may want to plan their funeral. Others may want to sign a living will that instructs doctors to discontinue life-support systems when there is no hope of survival. In most cases, there is ample time to make these preparations.

"All these things can be done to gain some control over death. And there's even more control. It's amazing. A study of several thousand deaths showed that almost 50 percent occurred within three months after people's birthdays, while fewer than 10 percent came in the three months before their birthdays."

"I don't understand the point," said the man.

"Just this," said the Cancer Conqueror. "People seem to have an influence over the time of death. Many 'postponed' their death until after they had celebrated another birthday."

"That's incredible," said the man. "Can we be certain?"

"No," said the Cancer Conqueror, "there isn't a certainty here. I'm not saying that we can live forever. But I am suggesting that we do have some degree of control that perhaps we once thought did not exist. And another point on control. I've been able to work with a team of professionals who, as part of an integrated cancer treatment plan, teach patients about death. The senior psychologist feels that there is strong evidence that many people die as they have lived."

"What does that mean?" asked the man.

"It's back again to this issue of fearing a low quality of death. The team observes that patients who live a life of anger may experience an 'angry' death. Conversely, those who live a life of love, joy, and peace nearly always reflect this in their death.

"Again, the lesson is to love. We can choose to love now, to be joyful now, and to make peace of mind real now. In short, we can choose to live fully as long as we live by showing love to ourselves and to those around us. The result: The quality of death is almost always a reflection of the quality of life. Very little time is spent actually dying; the time is spent living and loving as long as we are alive."

"I like that," said the man as he took a moment to ponder the point.

The man seemed touched by the hope in the Cancer Conqueror's message. There was a comfort in understanding that he could control the quality of his death by creating high quality in his life. And the idea of extending the reach of one's life by loving others unconditionally was most reassuring.

But after death, was he just a memory? That seemed less than fully satisfying. "What about life after death?" asked the man. "Do you think there is more to come after this life?"

Without hesitation the Cancer Conqueror answered, "To me the evidence is overwhelming. I believe that you and I are much more than physical bodies. I certainly do not pretend to know everything about this issue, yet I see so much evidence that death is the exit from this life and the entrance to the next plane of existence. To me, death doesn't have to be approached with fear. I think we can approach it with a healthy curiosity about what will be next. It can be viewed as a new adventure. Can you grasp that possibility?"

The man was deep in thought. Finally he looked at the

Cancer Conqueror and almost in a whisper asked, "There's comfort in those beliefs, isn't there?"

The Cancer Conqueror nodded. "For me there is. There's deep comfort and real hope. I believe there is much more that awaits me after life here on earth. But my concept of life, not death, is what makes the difference. This compels me to love now. The result is inner harmony and personal peace about whatever may be on the next plane."

The man stopped again. He was considering some of the implications of what the Cancer Conqueror was saying. "The next plane. Inner harmony. Personal peace. This almost has a mystical quality to it. Does the cancering journey become some sort of religious experience?"

"Some people would not be comfortable with the word *religious* or *mystical*. I prefer to use the term *spiritual* when we discuss this. And yes," said the Cancer Conqueror, "in my experience, cancering becomes very much a spiritual journey."

"Then please help me understand this part," said the man.

"Just consider the context," said the Cancer Conqueror. "We live in two worlds, the material and the spiritual. Most of our education, our effort, even our awareness is centered in the material. But consider the cancer journey. While there is certainly a material, physical element, we quickly move beyond it. We talk about beliefs that are positive, that serve our health well. Then we move on to resolve, managing the emotional conflict that can depress our mind and our body's immune response. And we make a decision to *live*. Those are all issues of the human spirit. The context of cancering has now become spiritual."

"John made that clear," said the man. "I understand the principles. But I sense I am missing a dimension. I sense this all leads somewhere."

"Excellent," said the Cancer Conqueror. "It certainly does lead somewhere. As you begin to choose the spiritual path, you'll also begin to recognize the breadth and depth of that choice. It pervades your entire life experience."

"That's good," said the man, "'pervades your entire life experience.' I feel that's what is happening to me right now. I sense that I am beginning to open to a whole new life. What is actually going on here?"

The Cancer Conqueror deliberated a moment. Was the man prepared for a more in-depth look at the spiritual road? Would he be able to grasp its dimensions and be ready for the implications of this choice? And could the Cancer Conqueror explain it in a way that would not alienate him? It was a pivotal moment. The Cancer Conqueror inched ahead.

"I can best explain this by starting once again with beliefs. This time the beliefs are not about the illness. They are about life. There are certain core convictions and foundational beliefs that profoundly affect our life experience in virtually every aspect. They do much to determine the quality of life on all levels. These core choices affect us far beyond our bodies, far beyond cancer."

"Okay," said the man, "what are they?"

"Perhaps the most fundamental belief relates to the essence of the world in which we live. For centuries, the greatest minds have debated the nature of the universe. Did biological accident or divine direction create our experience? In short, the first core belief asks the question, Is there a God?

"I encourage you to choose a healthy conviction here. I encourage you to believe that there is a God who knows us and loves us. And God loves us even though God knows us!"

❧❧

There is a God

who knows us and loves us.

And God loves us

even though

God knows us.

❧❧

"That's a healthy choice?" asked the man.

"Very healthy," said the Cancer Conqueror. "There are significant implications in that statement. Let's examine them. First, there is the choice that God really does exist and that God is part of our existence."

"Well, sometimes I'm not so sure," said the man.

The Cancer Conqueror smiled. "I can't show you a randomized double-blind study offering documented proof that there is a God. I can't take you down the street to a place of worship and say, 'See, look at God.' On this point, your personal beliefs are the determining factor."

"I don't know," said the man. "I'm not very comfortable with anything religious."

The Cancer Conqueror touched the man's arm. "Look, the last thing I want to do is make you uncomfortable. But I am not the one who is making you uncomfortable. You are making you uncomfortable."

"Okay," said the man. "But the fact remains, I just don't know that much about God."

"You do know that there is something outside yourself, don't you?" asked the Cancer Conqueror. "After all, you didn't make this world. And I didn't create the universe. Certainly there must be some kind of power outside you and me. Would you agree a greater intelligence is behind our existence?"

"Well, from that standpoint, there must be something," said the man. "But does that mean 'God'?"

"Perhaps you're letting the word *God* get in your way. To some people the word *God* is full of negative connotations, especially that of judgmentalism. In all the languages of the world, people use different names for the divine. The most widely used in the English language is *God*. For the moment, try to drop some of your previously learned concepts about God. Would you be able to explore the spiritual path openly for just a few minutes?"

"Okay," said the man. "I can do that."

"Good," said the Cancer Conqueror. "For the moment, just accept that there is 'something' that is a higher power. We call that power God. Let's look again at the core belief. There is a God who knows us and loves us, and God loves us even though God knows us. First, there is a primary conclusion, an affirmation, a conviction, that acknowledges a power behind our existence. There is a God of the world."

The Cancer Conqueror continued, "The second part of our core belief states that there is a God 'who knows us.' The implications of this statement are significant. Not only are we saying that there is a God but we are also affirming that this God is aware of you and me as individuals. You are known to God personally, by name, by thought, by spirit, by all the ways that God can identify and recognize us. This is no abstract power—this is a personal, one-on-one relationship with the central creative force behind everything that exists."

The man was thoughtful. Even though he didn't speak, the Cancer Conqueror could sense his attentiveness.

"Now take our core belief another step. The belief goes on to say, 'and God loves us.' Imagine that. The very power that created everything in existence knows and loves us! Wow!"

The man smiled at the Cancer Conqueror's enthusiasm. Perhaps this was something about which he could be enthusiastic. Whenever the man did think about God, he always envisioned some sort of mean judge. "A God of love," that was certainly more comforting.

The Cancer Conqueror went on. "Let's complete our look at the core belief. It ends by stating, 'and God loves us even though God know us.' This means that even when we don't perform to our potential, we are still loved. In the eyes of the creator of all, we are not what we do or don't do. We receive God's love simply because we are God's creation. God chooses to love us as we are!"

The man said, "But I don't see how this influences my cancer journey."

"All this acknowledges the fact that God is for us! God wants our total wellness. Our task is one of alignment, to become attuned with the messages cancer is sending us, to make the required changes, and to accept God's love and direction for our lives."

The man snapped, "How can that be? If God is for us, why did God give us cancer?"

The Cancer Conqueror paused and smiled that serene smile. She understood how critical her next words would be. "I don't believe God did give us cancer," she said. "My belief is that this illness is not God's will but is actually a deviation from God's will. In fact, I now believe that those things that bring sorrow, distress, calamity, and even suffering are ultimately present in the world not as God's will but as a result of our misunderstanding of God's will."

"Well, maybe," said the man, "but it seems to me that God at least allowed the cancer."

"Perhaps," said the Cancer Conqueror. "But even that is not the perspective you'll need to conquer cancer. The key is to understand the message. Grasp this. Cancer is really an opportunity, perhaps even God's direction, for us to change. I often think of cancer as a gift, a valuable opportunity to reshape life. And when I began to understand the depth of this truth, my whole thinking about God and life and cancer changed."

There was silence. The two looked squarely into each other's eyes. The man sat with clenched jaw, pondering the implications of what was being said. The Cancer Conqueror sent up a silent prayer, "Speak through me now, God," and then she continued.

"I've also come to understand that many people feel as if cancer is a sign that God let them down. It's a disappointment with, even an anger at, God. An extremely devout woman once said to me, 'When I was diagnosed with colon cancer, I felt God had totally let me down.'"

The man nodded. "I understand. I feel the same way. I've felt that way for years about God—in my business, in my relationships, in all areas of life. It all makes me doubt that God, if he or she is there, really cares for us."

The Cancer Conqueror often heard this set of spiritual questions, especially among people who were sincerely trying to do the work of wellness. She recognized the questioning as a healthy sign; these were positive doubts. "I've felt the same way," she said. "When I was first diagnosed, I thought, Hey God, I kept my part of the deal pretty well. Why didn't you keep your part of the deal?"

"That's exactly it," said the man. "That's just what I'm thinking."

"I've learned that when we start thinking that way," said the Cancer Conqueror, "it's actually pointing out that our model of the divine plan may not be accurate. From the experience of many cancer patients, I suggest you don't interpret cancer as a sign that God has abandoned you. Believe this. God does care for us, God will help us, now and in whatever lies in our future. What is required is a patient response that puts us back in touch with the message of cancer."

The man took careful notes. He was intuitively aware of the critical importance of what he had just heard. He would come back to these points later. The Cancer Conqueror was continuing.

"Focus on the message to change. Understanding the message in cancer brings us face-to-face with our second core belief. It has to do with the nature of our life experiences. There are many ways to say this. But the one that communicates best to me states, Life is a loving teacher.

❧❧

Life is a

loving teacher.

❧❧

"If God loves us," continued the Cancer Conqueror, "God will want the best for us. God will lovingly guide and direct our paths. Thus, through our life experiences—both pleasant and unpleasant—lessons are going to be taught."

"See," said the man, "this is the point. I have trouble believing that a God who is lovingly trying to teach us would be so cruel as to cause or even allow cancer. That's simply not loving."

"Now think," continued the Cancer Conqueror firmly, "of the consistency with the earlier belief that cancer is a process and a message to change. Some lessons that God lovingly gives, or even allows, are pleasant. Other lessons are anything but pleasant. Yet all teach, guide, and direct our lives. Perhaps there are times when we get so off the spiritual track that the only way God can gain our attention is through an event that is nearly catastrophic."

"This sounds like the vindictive, judge-type God that I was taught about as a child," said the man.

"Not so," countered the Cancer Conqueror. "God is not some unreasonable and impulsive sovereign. This is a loving God who has created a universe that runs by natural laws. This loving God doesn't give out punishment on a whim."

"But God is omnipotent," said the man. "God can do anything God wants to do."

"Certainly," said the Cancer Conqueror, "but also recognize that God has put in place the natural laws that run the world. And God seldom breaks those laws. They are the natural order of this world. It's healthy to believe that even cancer is a message for us to become more aligned with those spiritual laws. That is what all of life is trying to teach us—to become more aligned with God's will."

"That's hard for me to accept," said the man.

"Think of it this way then," said the Cancer Conqueror. "Illness and health send us messages, both negative and positive. Both messages tell us how we are doing. Health, happiness, peace, joy, and love are all intended as messages that we are doing well. Illness, and pain—both physical and psychological—depression, fear, and despair are all negative messages that are intended to bring us back on course. All are loving teachers."

The man shook his finger at the Cancer Conqueror. "But your philosophy is all wrong. The true nature of people is not good, it is evil. I can remember the exact words I was taught, 'Man is by nature sinful and unclean.' It doesn't make sense to have a loving God who is a loving teacher if people are inherently bad. These lessons you talk about would never get through. You need to punish evil. And I think God must use cancer as his chief means of punishment."

The Cancer Conqueror was dismayed. She recognized these were all learned beliefs and behavior, real roadblocks that had been constructed in the man's spiritual path. But at least they explained his attitudes.

"No, no, no!" she said. "Emphatically no! I don't like to confront you, but this is an important point. There is a better way. There are better beliefs! In fact, this is core belief number three—God created people in innocence and goodness.

"I went through this struggle," said the Cancer Conqueror. "I was taught that original sin left me totally helpless, that some people are predestined to live in eternal despair, and that my behavior could be controlled only with a heavy dose of fear and guilt. I was frightened by a God who was out to get me. Those beliefs are not true. They confuse what a person does with the way God creates. In point of fact, virtually all religions acknowledge that people are created in innocence and goodness. The concept of evil we hear so many people emphasize came later.

"When the emphasis is on *evil*, guilt almost always is the end result. This is sad and destructive. These teachings simply do not go deep enough. And worse, they inflict untold scars on people. It is my personal belief that many illnesses, including cancer, may be caused or prolonged because people condemn themselves and others with this guilt."

"I'm not sure what you're saying," said the man. "How does this apply to my getting well?"

The Cancer Conqueror continued, "Simply stated, if you believe, either consciously or subconsciously, that God created people as inherently evil, you will consider yourself unworthy. And unworthiness certainly is not the perspective of wellness."

"So then," said the man, "what is that wellness perspective?"

"I encourage you to hold firmly to the conviction that people, at the very core of their being, have unlimited potential for kindness, goodness, and gentleness—particularly as they connect with God's awesome presence. I also encourage you to believe in people's ability to love. Perhaps the message behind cancer is that God can change people! Perhaps the real message of cancer is threefold: Love God, love others, love ourselves."

"But there is so much evil out in the world. How can you say that people have the capacity for unlimited kindness, goodness, gentleness, and love? I think this is very much at odds with actual experience," said the man.

The Cancer Conqueror smiled. "Remember the central lesson of *live*—unconditional love?"

"Yes, I do," the man answered. "It was a huge leap in personal growth for me. But how does it apply here?"

"Let's review," said the Cancer Conqueror. "First we looked within to realize that we do not have some terrible central flaw in our being that makes us hopeless. Next we looked around and realized that others were just the same, and that we could learn to accept them as fellow human beings, even though we may not approve of their behavior. And finally we focused on our role—to be loving and forgiving without expecting anything in return."

"Yes, I know," said the man. "That liberated me. But I still don't see your point."

The Cancer Conqueror looked unwaveringly into the man's eyes. This would be a critical point. She shot up another prayer for guidance.

"Just as you have been liberated by extending unconditional love to yourself and to others, know that a loving God is extending even more and greater love to you."

The Cancer Conqueror paused for several seconds. "And even though our behavior may not always match our potential, even though our capacity for kindness, goodness, and gentleness is not fully realized, we can receive God's love because God loves us for who we are, not for what we do!"

Another long pause. "Because of God's great love, we are still acceptable even though we may be imperfect." She repeated, "You and I . . . we are imperfect but acceptable."

❧❧

We are imperfect but acceptable.

❧❧

The Cancer Conqueror just stopped and fixed her gaze directly on the man's eyes. The long silence was finally broken by the whisper of the man himself. "Imperfect but acceptable."

The Cancer Conqueror didn't say a word. She just nodded her head in agreement. Tears welled up in the man's eyes. She could sense a transformation under way.

The man sank back in his chair. "Nobody ever explained it like this before," he whispered. "A loving, personal God, the creator of all there is, life as a loving teacher, and people who are not rejected because of their imperfections.

"I'm not perfect, but I am acceptable. And I am loved," he continued in a hushed voice. "I can't tell you what this means to me." He paused again. "This is the first time in my life that I have experienced nonjudgmental, unconditional love."

The man stopped speaking. It was an emotional, pivotal moment.

Finally the Cancer Conqueror spoke. "This is a love that heals. Accept it. This love is the gateway to knowing personal peace. This love ultimately conquers cancer. And this love often cures it too."

More silence. The man was meditating. At last he asked, "There are no guarantees on this path, are there?"

"If you're looking for a sure cure on the purely physical level, nobody can offer you one with integrity. But on the spiritual level, the answer is right before you. You are known. You are loved. You are acceptable. Yes. It's guaranteed."

The two sat quietly. The man felt a sense of peacefulness that was completely new to him.

"I want to know more about the love of God," he said. "Where do I turn? Do I go back to church? Do I turn to religion? Do I pray day and night? What's next?"

The Cancer Conqueror smiled. "You may personally feel you need to do one or even all those things. That will be your decision. But start with the inner journey. Start with aligning yourself with God's love. Practice dispensing unconditional love without ceasing. It's the aligned spirit that God seeks."

"And then what?" asked the man.

"This will quickly bring you to a point of realization: You and I are completely dependent on God. Everything, including life and health and all provision, even every breath we draw, is another gift from God. When I became aware that God is my complete source," said the Cancer Conqueror, "I turned to the God of the scriptures. Here I discovered the special power of trusting in God's goodness that could be found nowhere else."

"This," said the man, "is the very point with which I have so much trouble. Can I really believe? Can I really trust this God?"

"Yes, you can," said the Cancer Conqueror. "You can trust God completely. But don't expect God to do it all for you. I want you to nurture trust in three physicians. Trust the physicians of the body, your medical team. Trust their competence and their integrity to do all you consent to on the physical level. Trust your inner physician, the inherent ability you possess to generate emotional harmony and physical healing. And trust the spiritual physician, the God who loves you and gives you true peace."

"Why not just pray for God to perform a miracle?" asked the man.

"God could," said the Cancer Conqueror. "We certainly want to allow for that. And God sometimes does that. But the natural laws by which God governs are seldom broken. Law-of-nature-defying miracles are certainly the exception. But law-of-nature-consistent miracles are happening every day. You elicit them when you trust and align with God's will. God is not lessened because of that. Believing in our own healing potential only acknowledges our true spiritual nature."

Both were quiet as they let these insights saturate their spirits. There was a vital power for living here. Finally the man said, "You know, I have a sense of calm—of deep peace—right now. I've never experienced this before. This is entirely new to me. In fact, I sense it's a new me."

The Cancer Conqueror smiled. This was the place she had hoped to bring the man.

"Peace is the goal," she said softly. "Knowing God's peace, even if we have cancer, that's what it means to conquer the illness.

"Our goal is peace with ourselves, with others, and with God. That goal is achieved by implementing the very things you have studied in your journey—believe, resolve, and *live!*

❧❧

Our goal is peace with ourselves, with others, and with God.

❧❧

"When the goal of peace is achieved, it may be temporary. In fact, try not to relate peace to time at all. It may be difficult to achieve peacefulness for more than a few minutes at a time. If so, don't be discouraged. It is the journey, not just the destination, that is the aim."

"I think I've heard that principle elsewhere," said the man. "Is that why everyone keeps referring to the 'cancer journey'?"

"Exactly," said the Cancer Conqueror. "It's a journey in search of God's peace. And the sooner you make it a *live* journey, the sooner you will benefit from the lessons and come to experience you own peace."

She continued, "Now consider this. If cancer is a message to change, what is it you are called to be . . . and to do? Put the emphasis here on *called*."

"What do you mean?" asked the man.

"Just this. Cancer is asking you to change. It's a call toward a new life. You are called to be someone. You are called to do something. You are being called into a transformation. Pursue that call. Within it will be your reason for living.

"Don't be driven," continued the Cancer Conqueror. "Be *called*. Take the time to listen and respond to the call."

"That call," asked the man, "is it centered in loving and helping others?"

"You know it is!" said the Cancer Conqueror. "Your call will take the form of love toward self, love toward others, and love toward God. And you'll know you are succeeding when what you think, what you say, and what you do are consistent with God's directions."

Again the two sat in silence. There was a deep peacefulness in their presence. The Cancer Conqueror prayed. The man was listening to that call from within.

Finally the Cancer Conqueror spoke again. "The achieving is in the doing. Go and do."

There was another silence. Then the two stood and embraced. And the man left silently. God's peace was with him.

❦ Author's Encouragement ❦

Our story continues on page 215. However, I ask you to explore some of your spiritual beliefs now. Please take a moment to appreciate the majesty of your awesome divine connection.

❧ TRANSCEND: ❧
ATTAINING SPIRITUAL CONNECTION

Your spirit, that immaterial and vital intelligence that animates you, is incredibly powerful. Optimal health and well-being is the by-product of your physical, mental, emotional, and spiritual factors. Yet spirit is often the most misunderstood and least utilized of our considerable healing resources. Spirit is much more than a mere resource; it is our very essence. All of us are spiritual beings. We are "chips off the divine block." To be spiritual implies a conscious awareness of that power that is our ultimate nature, as well as a conscious connection with a dimension of vital intelligence that is greater than ourselves. Awareness of our connection—this is the key.

Spirituality is founded on a recognition that life is sacred and has been given to us as a gift. The fact that cancer may temporarily obscure a portion of this gift in no way diminishes its priceless value.

It is easy to lose sight of the spiritual component of life. We struggle with cancer, forgetting that pain can be an opportunity for spiritual awakening. We hope the wonders of modern medicine will restore our vitality. Yet we forget that the root definition of health is wholeness, which includes mending the spirit.

One of the most significant redeeming opportunities of cancer is that we are given ample favorable circumstances to discover the transcendent dimension of life: Is there a God? What is my life's meaning? What am I on this earth to accomplish? In a decade and a half of working personally with over fifteen thousand cancer patients, I can report without equivocation that nurturing a deeper spirituality is central to healing. It is awesome and predictable; when people move beyond medical care, diet, exercise, stress management, they invariably come to the journey of the soul. It is often a turning point, for this is the terrain of healing. It is also virgin territory for most people. Cancer has brought them to the frontier of their existence. The conversations typically turn quiet and serious, as if we had crossed a threshold into the most tender and sacred aspects of life.

I have been exceedingly fortunate to be a healing guide to many people and have witnessed a wide variety of intimate spiritual experiences. I can report that one size does not fit all. Some people have "reflex" spiritual answers: "I turned my troubles over to God and decided to live to be a hundred." Or, "I just let go and let God." For many others spirituality is an introduction to humility. A powerful business executive, diagnosed with metastatic prostate cancer, shook his head and quietly said, "When I realized this situation was out of my control, the only comfort I had was a belief in the ultimate goodness of God."

The portals of healing can be opened in many ways. Religious orientation is less the deciding factor than a conscious awareness of a personal, reciprocal, loving connection with the divine. Ponder thoughtfully the words *conscious, awareness, personal, reciprocal, loving, connection.* I am persuaded that this type of spiritual transcendence, over time, has demonstrated power to help people heal. At the least, it is central to recovering a sense of balance, tranquillity, and hope. And, as I have both experienced and observed, those states of spirit are very often prerequisites for a cure.

Whether it is a fundamentalist's fervent belief in the power of prayer or an agnostic's deep reverence for life, I have come to understand there is nothing in medicine that equals the power of standing consciously in the awesome presence of God.

Awaken Your Spirit

Consider each statement. Indicate your level of agreement by circling the relative value from 10 to 1, 10 indicating that you strongly agree, 1 that you strongly disagree. Reflect on your level of intensity surrounding each belief.

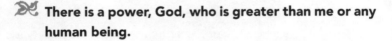 **There is a power, God, who is greater than me or any human being.**

Strongly agree		Somewhat agree		Not certain either way		Somewhat disagree		Strongly disagree	
10	9	8	7	6	5	4	3	2	1

Thought Starters: Am I comfortable calling that greater power God? If not, what name do I use? In what specific ways is God more powerful than I am?

_____

_____

_____

_____

_____

_____

_____

_____

_____

_____

_____

_____

_____

_____

❧ God knows me personally, both "who" and "what" I am.

Strongly agree		Somewhat agree		Not certain either way		Somewhat disagree		Strongly disagree	
10	9	8	7	6	5	4	3	2	1

Thought Starters: What are three titles that define "who" I am? (for example, mother, father, homemaker, lawyer). At my essence, "what" am I? Would changing my "who" change my "what"? How about vice versa?

_____

_____

_____

_____

_____

_____

_____

_____

_____

_____

_____

_____

_____

_____

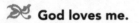 **God loves me.**

Strongly agree		Somewhat agree		Not certain either way		Somewhat disagree		Strongly disagree	
10	9	8	7	6	5	4	3	2	1

Thought Starters: Respond to the idea "God believes in you. God wants the best (health) for you." What does your thoughtful answer reveal about your concept of God?

_____

_____

_____

_____

_____

_____

_____

_____

_____

_____

_____

_____

_____

_____

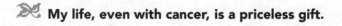 **My life, even with cancer, is a priceless gift.**

Strongly agree		Somewhat agree		Not certain either way		Somewhat disagree		Strongly disagree	
10	9	8	7	6	5	4	3	2	1

Thought Starters: Respond to the idea "A gift implies a giver and requires a response of gratitude." What has cancer taught you about thankfulness?

_____

_____

_____

_____

_____

_____

_____

_____

_____

_____

_____

_____

_____

❧ My death will be an exit from this life and an entrance into my next level of experience.

Strongly agree		Somewhat agree		Not certain either way		Somewhat disagree		Strongly disagree	
10	9	8	7	6	5	4	3	2	1

Thought Starters: What are my thoughts and feelings about the process of dying? About severing my earthly relationships?

_____

_____

_____

_____

_____

_____

_____

_____

_____

_____

_____

_____

❧ I can significantly control my quality of death by focusing on my quality of my life.

Strongly agree		Somewhat agree		Not certain either way		Somewhat disagree		Strongly disagree
10	9	8	7	6	5	4	3	2	1

Thought Starters: List three ways you should then live. Follow each with an action point that would immediately improve your life quality.

_____

_____

_____

_____

_____

_____

_____

_____

_____

_____

_____

_____

_____

_____

_____

_____

I am open to the lessons of my pain and grief.

Strongly agree		Somewhat agree		Not certain either way		Somewhat disagree		Strongly disagree
10	9	8	7	6	5	4	3	2	1

Thought Starter: Describe what have you learned about God, life, and yourself in the darkness of cancer.

_____

_____

_____

_____

_____

_____

_____

_____

_____

_____

_____

_____

_____

_____

_____

_____

❧ I have weighed my options and have decided to pre-pare to live.

Strongly agree		Somewhat agree		Not certain either way		Somewhat disagree		Strongly disagree	
10	9	8	7	6	5	4	3	2	1

Thought Starters: List the commitments you must make to begin the process of regaining your health. Or to begin the process of accepting death.

_____

_____

_____

_____

_____

_____

_____

_____

_____

_____

_____

_____

_____

_____

_____

❧ I love others and know that I am loved by others.

Strongly agree		Somewhat agree		Not certain either way		Somewhat disagree		Strongly disagree	
10	9	8	7	6	5	4	3	2	1

Thought Starters: Who do you love? Who loves you? Who will cherish you in their memories? Is this a factor you wish to improve upon—starting now?

_____

_____

_____

_____

_____

_____

_____

_____

_____

_____

_____

_____

_____

_____

❧ I understand that knowing God's peace is my goal and that well-being is the by-product.

Strongly agree		Somewhat agree		Not certain either way		Somewhat disagree		Strongly disagree	
10	9	8	7	6	5	4	3	2	1

Thought Starters: Describe what you understand to be the signs of God's peace. Are they present in your life? How can you cultivate greater peace?

_____

_____

_____

_____

_____

_____

_____

_____

_____

_____

_____

_____

_____

_____

For the Advanced Wellness Student

Experiencing and expressing a transcendent spirituality is an intentional choice. We do not have to entertain nagging suggestions about what the future may hold. Fear, uncertainty, and ambivalence need not paralyze us in living. Instead, we can choose to live in the spiritual bliss of forgiveness, gratitude, and unconditional love.

Focusing on the moment may seem like classic denial, especially for those with cancer. Unless it is a mindless reaction, however, such focusing is not denial.

Spirit does transcend. It may be difficult to believe that this is the best time of your life. Cancer colors so much of the lens through which we see our experiences. The view can seem dark and foreboding, as if a storm of epic proportions is on the horizon. Yet this is the best time of your life because it is the only time of your life. Nothing else exists but the eternal now. In the spiritual realm, yesterday and tomorrow are simply an illusion. God and all things good are eternally present.

You have a choice: You can choose to align with God and all that is good, or you can choose to bring the past and the future into this moment. Transcendent spirits align with the good in this moment.

You seek to change the pattern of your physical health. The only moment in which this can be accomplished is the now. To do so is, ultimately, a spiritual experience. This is a big order but not impossible.

So you and I must be ever vigilant to create healing. Are you treating this moment, as you read these very lines, as a brand-new moment for well-being? How can you make it new and precious and filled with health? Respond to the following query:

🐝 **How can I express spiritual well-being, in this "now" moment? List as many ways as you can.**

_____

_____

_____

_____

_____

_____

_____

_____

_____

_____

_____

_____

Two of our most powerful tools for spiritual transcendence are the power found in silence and the power of the spoken word. Our spoken word can become an affirmative claim on divine substance. Our word begins to materialize what we want and what God wants for us. Our word is how we think about and relate to God and God's will.

The first verse of the Twenty-third Psalm is not only the best-known of all the Psalms but also, based on my observations, the most widely used health affirmation on earth. People of all faiths, people with no faith, constantly call on its healing, calming influence:

The Lord is my shepherd; I shall not want.

I have seen this simple affirmation help people calm fears, center in the moment, align with God, and begin the healing process. This affirmation embodies healing as it connects us to our spiritual essence.

The Awe and Wonder of Healing

A dramatic demonstration of the healing potential of the Twenty-third Psalm came as our Cancer Recovery Retreat team welcomed a gentleman named Victor to one of our programs. He had metastatic liver cancer. Too weak to walk, Victor checked in to the retreat center in a wheelchair. His breathing was labored; an oxygen tank was strapped to the back of his chair, and the tubes from the tank led to his nostrils. A persistent hiss could be heard from the apparatus.

Victor's skin color was ashen. He was dressed in a dark blue athletic warm-up jacket over a sweatshirt and wrapped in a heavy wool stadium blanket; he complained of having been cold ever since his chemotherapy. Victor's voice was a weak and raspy whisper. He coughed often. I believed he was very close to death.

Because of his obvious need, we suspended our normal first-evening orientation and concentrated on ministering to him. After about thirty minutes of faltering attempts at communication, one of the counselors asked, "Victor, do you have a favorite verse of scripture?" His labored reply was, "The Lord is my shepherd. I shall not want."

In what I can only describe as a divinely inspired response, the entire group of counselors, fellow patients, and family support members—about thirty people in all—gathered around Victor, laying hands on his head, shoulders, and arms. We began to reverently repeat his favorite verse, "The Lord is my shepherd. I shall not want."

At first, Victor had no response. But the affirmations continued, quietly, reverently, simply, person after person, "The Lord is my shepherd. I shall not want."

Victor finally responded, silently nodding his head in agreement.

Then someone in the group said, "The Lord is my physician. I shall not want." And that was soon followed by, "The Lord is my healer. I shall not want." The tone became more positively expectant.

Victor managed to respond with a whispered yes.

One of the other participants then said, "The Lord is my treatment. I shall not want." Someone else followed with "The Lord is my source, I shall not want." And another voice affirmed, "The Lord is my health. I shall *never* want."

Victor's posture became more upright; he grew more alert. He smiled and said with a clearer and stronger voice, "I shall *never* want." You could discern the emphasis he placed on the word *never*.

As these affirmations, all derived from the first sentences of the Twenty-third Psalm, continued, we experienced what I can only call a miracle, actually several miracles. A woman participant, who we later learned was suffering with painful neuropathy following chemotherapy, began to weep uncontrollably. She sobbed, then moaned. She collapsed to the floor and was held by another woman, who simply kept repeating, "The Lord is our shepherd. We shall not want." The moaning continued; it was painful just to hear the sounds that originated from deep within the woman's body and spirit.

Victor's color seemed to be improving.

Another woman, wearing a turban that covered her chemotherapy-induced baldness, stood with hands stretched over her head and began repeating, "Lord, you are my healing. I shall never want." Soon a group of five or six were gathered around her, hands held upward, affirming with her, "Lord, you are my healing. I shall never want."

Victor unwrapped himself from the blanket. He was perspiring.

I hesitate to report this event because I am deeply suspicious of healing theatrics. Yet, as much as I did not, and still do not, seek this type of emotionalism, something otherworldly was obviously at work here.

Victor leaned forward, then stood up, directly in front of his wheelchair. He was tall and thin, yet he now had a whole new persona. And in one of only two times I have seen a personal aura—the luminous energy field that is believed to emanate from all living beings—Victor was surrounded by a glowing light.

I stood back in awe, even fear, and watched the light around Victor change from purple to orange to golden yellow to bright white. I was later to learn that I was one of only two people who saw it. Not even Victor realized its presence. It disturbed me that everyone did not see it. Was I hallucinating? I can only report it was very real.

The large room became silent. The woman who had been sobbing and moaning was now quiet, her energy spent. She was held and prayed for by several people. The group that surrounded the turban-clad woman was now embraced in a huddle of fifteen or more. Several of us just stood by in wonder.

It was Victor who finally spoke. "I think I have been healed."

That was nearly four years ago. Victor is alive and well. The woman with neuropathy is pain-free. The woman in the turban now works with us in Southern California.

I do not pretend to fully understand what happened that evening. And in the few occasions I have shared this experience with others who claim to be experts in this field, the explanations leave me wanting. Victor, in his annual Hanukkah letter, referred to it briefly by saying, "When I acknowledged God as my complete source, I was healed."

I understand that explanation. It is present in many healing experiences.

I also understand that we have an incomplete knowledge of healing. Experiences like this defy modern science and certainly challenge conventional thinking. Yet they are integral to the lives of thousands of people who are healed. Unlike a decade ago, now I welcome the fact that we are able to share these experiences without the fear of clinical dismissal or theological condemnation.

This I also understand. There is a power within us. It is within you just as surely as it is within me. I believe this power is responsive to our highest needs. When we make conscious connection with this power, it literally transforms our lives, because in our true nature we are this power in expression.

You and I live by and in the gift of God's goodness. We do not have to entertain the nagging thoughts of fear that create dis-ease. Even in the midst of cancer, especially in the midst of cancer, I encourage you to acknowledge God as your complete source. Become consciously aware of that powerful connection. Therein is found God's peace. Therein is healing of the highest order.

Cancer
Conquerors Share

A s the weeks passed, the man put to use what he had learned. And guess what happened? He became a Cancer Conqueror! It happened not just because the man talked like a Cancer Conqueror but because he had learned a better way to *live*. And as the weeks built into months, he realized that it was not simply that he had learned new skills and knowledge but that he implemented what he had learned. This was a better life. Cancer really was a signal to change. New freedom was his! Love, joy, and peace were real to him!

At the end of the first year, the man looked back to the day when he had first met the Caner Conqueror. Since that time he had changed so much. His beliefs about cancer were radically different. He had resolved some fundamental issues he hadn't even recognized before the cancer.

And choosing to *live* had given him a freedom of spirit previously unimaginable.

The man was thrilled to understand for the first time in his life that he really was the one in control. But it was a spiritual control, one unlike most people sought, for certainly the man was not the ultimate power. Nor was he immune to all the problems life offered. Rather, the man had now developed a new power over himself, a power within, that allowed him to choose how to respond to the events of life. Daily he aligned himself with God's will, recognizing this was his complete source of power and control. This was living! This was conquering cancer!

The man began sharing his journey with newly diagnosed patients. It was most encouraging to see people change their beliefs, resolve emotional conflicts, then choose to *live*. The man made himself more and more available for these times of sharing. Cancer had taught him some valuable lessons. He was becoming a student of life, and at the same time he was becoming a teacher of living. He greatly enjoyed helping others learn to help themselves.

Perhaps what he enjoyed most, though, was the mastery over his own life. Every day, in every way, he was learning to *live*. He felt fully capable of dealing with today in a way that helped others as he helped himself and the world in which he lived.

The phone rang.

A young woman introduced herself. She explained that she had just been diagnosed with cancer. "I have been told that I have a journey ahead of me. I know I have a lot to learn. I would like to learn from the best. May I come talk to you?"

The man smiled that serene smile he had seen so many times before. Now he realized the smile was a sign that all was well—very well! It felt so good to be in this position. He had learned a great deal. He was one of the most significant success stories because he had come from despair to hope. Now he knew inner peace—God's peace.

"Of course you can come talk with me," he answered.

As soon as the young woman arrived, he began the conversation. "I'm happy to share my experiences with you. In doing so, I have just one request."

"What is that?" she asked.

"That you share this hope with others!"

❦❧

Share this hope

with others.

❦❧

❧ *Epilogue* ❧

Connection with spirit is often not found through religious practice. Yet the religious beliefs we hold greatly influence our approach to and experience of spiritual connection.

I offer you two closing thoughts on establishing this connection. First, honor the existing core beliefs you bring. Often these have roots in the faith of your youth. Spiritual paradigm changes frequently lead, in the short term, to increased emotional uncertainty, something you need less of at this moment. I suggest you make your connection through the religious faith you now practice.

The second thought is a caution: Beware of ritual. To be sure, religious ritual can give comfort; it has a place for many people. But spiritual connection goes far beyond comfort; it is a living, breathing, dynamic force and power.

You can sense the presence in all the ways God reveals healing. My observation, confirmed by hundreds of other people's experiences, is that spiritual connections are seldom established through ceremony or social custom.

I encourage you to travel this path. Integrate body, mind, and spirit. The journey leads to well-being—on the highest level.

I wish you blessings on your journey.

❧ Notes ❧

✂ Notes ✂

Notes

Notes

❈ *Notes* ❈

❧ ABOUT THE AUTHOR ❧

Greg Anderson is the author of six other books, including the international best-seller *The Cancer Conqueror*. His writings have been translated into eighteen languages.

Greg Anderson received his wake-up call in 1984. It was in the form of lung cancer. Four months after a lung was removed, the cancer metastasized through his lymph system. In December of that year, Anderson was told by his medical team he had just thirty days to live.

Contacting survivors across North America, he conducted interviews with patients who were "supposed to die" but had lived. His question: Were there common characteristics of survivorship he could apply to his own search? Anderson found healing in the combination of body, mind, and spirit—the power of intentional lifestyle choices coupled with conventional medical care.

In 1985 he founded the organization that would become the Cancer Recovery Foundation of America, a nonprofit educational and support organization whose mission is to educate, empower, and encourage cancer patients regarding the full spectrum of treatment and recovery options. Anderson's work emphasizes the integration of the mental, emotional, and spiritual aspects of healing with traditional medical care.

Greg Anderson can be reached on the World Wide Web at http://www.CancerRecovery.org or through the Cancer Recovery Foundation of America's toll-free number, 1-800-238-6479, or by writing to P.O. Box 238, Hershey, PA 17033, USA.